# THE PERFORMANCE NUTRITIONIST

## VOL. 2

Further insights, reflections and advice
from practitioners working in elite sport

**DR JAMES C. MOREHEN**

Copyright © 2024 by Dr James C. Morehen. All rights reserved.

This book or any portion thereof may not be reproduced or used in any manner whatsoever without the express written permission of the publisher except for the use of brief quotations in a book review.

Cover image by: U.T Designs
Book design by: SWATT Books Ltd

Printed in the United Kingdom
First Printing, 2024

ISBN: 978-1-7398718-2-6 (Paperback)
ISBN: 978-1-7398718-3-3 (eBook)

Dr James C. Morehen
Bicester, Oxforshire

morehenperformance.com

# CONTENTS

Acknowledgements — 5
Dedication — 7
Foreword — 9
Introduction — 11

**CHAPTER 1:** Dr Trent Stellingwerff — 17

**CHAPTER 2:** Dr David Dunne — 39

**CHAPTER 3:** Ted Munson — 53

**CHAPTER 4:** Charles Ashford — 73

**CHAPTER 5:** Ruth Wood-Martin — 95

**CHAPTER 6:** Lauren Delany — 113

**CHAPTER 7:** James Moran — 133

**CHAPTER 8:** Professor Louise Burke — 155

**CHAPTER 9:** Dr Dana Lis — 173

| | | |
|---|---|---|
| **CHAPTER 10:** | Mohamed Saad | *193* |
| **CONCLUSION:** | How To Stand Out From The Crowd | *211* |
| | Find Out More About the Performance Nutrition Network | *215* |
| | Mentorship Moments Course | *217* |
| | Recommended Resources | *221* |
| | About the Author | *225* |

# ACKNOWLEDGEMENTS

I would like to take this moment to thank three groups of people, my family, the interviewees, and the sport nutrition industry.

To my family, although I have many crazy ideas, they always support me with them and encourage me to finish what I start. Although I wanted this book to be published sooner, I have enjoyed spending time on developing me and growing up as a person. Nura and I got married, we welcomed our first child Mila to the world and have done a fair bit of travelling. A massive thank you to Nura and Mila for reminding me every day why I do what I do. To my brothers Daniel and Stephen for being the ears I need for my crazy but fulfilling ideas! Finally, my mother for just being Mother Hen; her strength over recent years following the loss of our dad and her husband reminds me that when life gets a little bit tough, we all have the fight in us to wake up tomorrow in a better place!

To Trent Stellingwerff, David Dunne, Ted Munson, Charles Ashford, Ruth Wood-Martin, Lauren Delany, James Moran, Louise Burke, Dana Lis and Mohamed Saad. Without you all dedicating time out of your busy lives to spend with me, this book could not be published. Each one of you provides nuggets of wisdom, advice and a wealth of craft knowledge which will inspire hundreds of practitioners, researchers and academics around the globe. It is this knowledge exchange which will keep developing our industry forward and pushing the boundaries of how performance nutrition can play its part in world-class winning performances.

To the sport nutrition industry. I love what I do. The more I read into self-development, entrepreneurship and business, the more passion I develop to continue doing what I do. I thoroughly enjoy and get so much from mentoring and helping others develop. I get so excited in supporting athletes with evidence-based performance nutrition strategies which help winning performances. To the hundreds of people who purchased this book, thank you! You motivated me to write it and as with the mentoring, the performance nutrition network and my online courses, your support is always appreciated.

Without the sport nutrition industry, this book could not be written.
**James**

# DEDICATION

I dedicate this book to Nura, Mila, my mum, my brothers, and my dad.

> *"People rarely succeed, unless they are having fun in what they are doing."*
> Dale Carnegie

# FOREWORD

We often say, "It's not about us. We're just here to help our athletes go faster, higher, stronger." But from time to time, it's important to remember that it is also about us – at least if we want to grow as people, practitioners and mentors. How do we get to be our best selves? How can evolution and self-improvement allow us to be more effective in our work? What can we learn from others that we can incorporate into our personal or professional toolbox? Alternatively, is there anything that doesn't feel right or acts as a Cautionary Tale of what not to do?

As I move towards the last phases of my own career, I've had time to reflect on my own path. Sometimes, it was a sad and brutal experience. Things didn't work out in my Dream Job at the AIS. What now? At other times, like talking with James, a skilled interviewer and curious colleague, for this book, it was an uplifting experience that provided worthwhile and sometimes unexpected insights. Turns out there's lots to learn from my younger self who had no idea how to create a career that was fulfilling, pays the bills and leaves a legacy. But there are also new questions to ponder. How can I use the rest of my time to finish up any outstanding projects or unfulfilled dreams? What tips can I pass on to other people who would like to be performance nutritionists? Have I remembered to thank the people who were instrumental in my journey?

I love hearing about the journeys of fellow performance nutritionists. We're like snowflakes; none of us are the same. I didn't get to read the other chapters in this book before writing this foreword. But as I look at the list, I recognise close colleagues as well as people I have admired but haven't met. I'm eager to delve into their stories and reflections. I am sure all of them will have experienced twists and turns, and collected gems that generosity and bravery will allow them to share with us.

I thank James for the initiative that made this book happen, and for the readers of book 1 who created the momentum for the second volume. I congratulate new readers for recognising a good investment of time and cash. I'm positive you'll be rewarded – including wisdom that you didn't even know you needed!

**Professor Louise Burke**

# INTRODUCTION

Hello and welcome back to *The Performance Nutritionist*. I don't want to waste your time or the pages of this book taking you through the start of my own career path or journey again. If you want to know that then read the start of book 1, reach out to me, or listen to a few podcasts I have done this year and you will know my story.

One theme that hopefully came across in book 1 was how everyone has their own story. We all go on our own journeys and paths to the job roles we are in. Some paths last a few months or even a few years. For example, I spent four years with England football before my own path changed.

Since publishing *The Performance Nutritionist* version 1, my own career has shifted. I am now the lead performance nutritionist with Bristol Bears Rugby who play in the premiership division for rugby union here in the UK. Alongside this, I spent 18 months with England Rugby and the Red Roses where I supported the team in winning two back-to-back Grand Slam titles and becoming runners-up in the Women's Rugby World Cup in New Zealand in 2022, losing very narrowly in the final minutes of the match. I love my work in rugby and have a superb team of practitioners and colleagues at Bristol Bears including all the athletic performance coaches and chefs. If I am honest, it is the most aligned my nutrition vision has been with other departments and it is a pleasure to work at Bears with the calibre of players we have.

My own academic career (19 publications, 6 as lead and 13 as co-author) and importantly business are growing nicely. With better systems and processes involved, I have also made the most of a great book titled *Who Not How* (Dan Sullivan) and have since employed four individuals on contractual hours to help me grow Morehen Performance Ltd.

Early in 2023 I drafted plans for a global online community for performance nutritionists, dietitians and athlete support personnel. In June 2023, I launched **The Performance Nutrition Network** which has been such a fun project to be leading on. It is a community which is growing from strength to strength in terms of members (100+ and climbing each week), the amount of knowledge, tools and resources being shared and just the willingness and openness of practitioners to help each other out with their own careers and projects. It really is inspiring and warming to see so many people coming together to support each other in their own journeys to becoming better practitioners and more skilled business owners. Below is an extract taken from the welcome page within the community:

> *I specifically designed this community to mentor nutrition coaches who are keen to advance their careers. Our network thrives on a symbiotic relationship where mentorship is central – offering invaluable resources, insights, and one-on-one guidance from seasoned professionals in the field of performance nutrition. Whether you're looking to refine your coaching techniques, delve deeper into scientific research, or understand the nuances of athlete engagement, our collective expertise is here to assist you in reaching your professional aspirations.*
>
> *I believe that mentorship is not a one-way street but a collaborative effort that benefits all. As members, you will not only receive guidance but are also encouraged to share your own experiences, challenges, and successes. This creates a cycle of continuous learning and improvement for everyone involved. Your active participation enriches the community, turning it into a dynamic and invaluable hub for career development in the realm of performance nutrition.*

I decided to write a second version of *The Performance Nutritionist* because of you, the reader. The feedback I received from version 1 was overwhelmingly positive. You enjoyed the book and many left Amazon reviews or messaged me privately to express thanks for me publishing it. This also acted as a slight nudge for me to get the wheels in motion for the second book. I think we all agree that there are many superb researchers and practitioners working in sport and so it made sense for version 2 to be completed.

The first book was an idea I had during COVID, and I had the time to get the idea into a physical book which I could make available to you all. The second book has taken a little longer than I would have liked but that's mainly due to family life (I now have a daughter) and my own applied work and business growing.

In book 1 I interviewed, and you read about:

1. Craig Umenyi
2. Dr Lloyd Parker
3. Dr Daniel Martin
4. Hannah Sheridan
5. Dr Marcus Hannon
6. Dr Emma Tester
7. Dr Jill Leckey
8. Dr Chris Rosimus
9. Emma Gardner
10. Professor James Morton

Some of my own reflections and main learnings from this book were:

Be resilient, enjoy the lessons in your career, fact versus opinion, the whole world eats food, expectation of athlete knowledge, become someone who loves to read, learn how to be a great coach, don't be a d\*\*k head, be comfortable in asking, volunteer, become a deal master, pick the low hanging fruit first, what is your unique selling point, learn the Dunning Kruger model and finally enjoy being a part of a multi-disciplinary team.

In book 2 I have continued the global span of interviews from academics and practitioners across the world and various backgrounds. All work in sport to some capacity and many also run their own businesses or private practice. You will read my interviews with:

1. Dr Trent Stellingwerff
2. Dr David Dunne
3. Ted Munson
4. Charles Ashford
5. Ruth Wood-Martin
6. Lauren Delany
7. James Moran
8. Professor Louise Burke
9. Dr Dana Lis
10. Mohamed Saad

Although most research papers in sport nutrition have been published in the last 15 to 20 years, sport nutrition and dietetics continue to be one of the most popular and fasting growing careers in sport science. As a result, there are hundreds if not thousands of students graduating each year, some of whom believe having a snazzy Instagram account and lots of followers is the way to pave a career in this industry. Don't get me wrong, utilising one of the world's best free advertisement machines does help, but your Instagram account is not the marker which decides on your level of education, knowledge and ability to work with clients. Additionally, employers in sport aren't that bothered by it, 1-1 clients maybe, but not sport.

If you are reading this book and have your own business in sport nutrition or dietetics, then you will enjoy these chapters. I think more so than ever, with the impact of online coaching, the ability to coach anyone in the world and now artificial intelligence tools, it makes sense for many to operate their own businesses. During the interviews for these 10 individuals, I made plenty of notes for my own practice and business and I am confident as you work your way through the book that you will also have many light bulb moments for your own business.

I hope by the end of this you will agree that we have moved the needle forward and continued our journey of interviewing some of the world's best performance nutritionists who work both in sport and academia.

I will take this opportunity to remind you of The Performance Nutrition Network and mentorship programme that I run. If you are interested in knowing more about The Performance Nutrition Network, scan the QR code below:

As someone who enjoys growth and development, any feedback on this book is welcomed; please message me on Instagram or LinkedIn, or directly if you have my number. The only way I can get better is through feedback from you.

Finally, if you like this book and would be willing to spend two minutes on providing me with an Amazon review, I would be hugely thankful. I read every one of them and it also helps drive the book into the top 10 books in its genre.

Enjoy and speak soon.
**James**

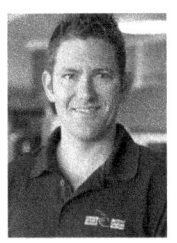

# CHAPTER 1:
# *DR TRENT STELLINGWERFF*

Trent is the director of performance solutions / applied sport research at Canadian Sport Institute Pacific.

I think the first time I met Trent in person was at the European College of Sport Science in either Malmo, Sweden or Dublin, Ireland. As a young nutrition student, I had read lots of Trent's research and admired his thirst for applied publications, none more so than the case study on his wife who at the time was a competitive athletics runner for Team Canada. If you want to read this case study, it is titled: "Case Study: Body Composition Periodization in an Olympic-Level Female Middle-Distance Runner Over a 9-Year Career".

I have also listened to Trent speak many times on podcasts and YouTube videos. With Trent's engaging personality, warming conversations and immense passion in the industry for applied performance and research (over 125 publications), it was both a privilege and a no-brainer to interview Trent for this book.

You can follow Trent on:
Twitter @TStellingwerff

**James Morehen: Let's begin with who you are and your background.**[1]

**Trent:** I'm Trent Stellingwerff, one of the directors of performance at the Canadian Sport Institute Pacific, one of our Olympic training centres in Canada. There are five across Canada, and we're out in beautiful British Columbia. I'm at our largest facility and headquarters in Victoria, and it's mainly a summer sports facility, and I've been here for 10 years. I have had a long and assorted journey to get here in Canada!

I am Canadian, and I grew up about 200 kilometres east near Toronto. I have two young boys at home, and doing it all with the travel demands was challenging. I've worked in various sports over the last 10 years; I was the lead physiologist for Rowing Canada, I've consulted with Triathlon Canada and Cycling Canada and for the previous seven years was the sports science medicine director for Athletics Canada, the governing body of Track and Field. Very recently, after a tremendous and incredible seven years, including a very successful Tokyo Olympics, with six medals for Athletics Canada, which was the best haul since the 1930s, I've transitioned out of that sport science medicine director role as it was just massive.

However, I'm still working at the Canadian Sport Institute, but now as the research and development lead for all of our projects and our strategy around innovation, research and development within our sports.

**We see your name in publication after publication, podcasts and being involved in an unbelievable amount of research projects. If you go back through your career, where was the first initial exposure or experience to what we call performance or sports nutrition?**

**Trent:** I come from a town of 600 people called Grand Bend, Ontario. My dad was a mechanic; he owned a garage, and my mom did the bookkeeping. No one from my family went to university. That being said, academics came relatively easy for me; I worked hard at it, but it came easy. Also, I was a decent runner, so I got a scholarship to go to the US to Cornell University, an Ivy League school.

---

[1] My questions and comments are in bold throughout the interview chapters.

I was undeclared (not yet decided or declared a major to study) when I started there as a major, but I took nutrition during my first year. As everyone said, it's a great course with a great teacher. I remember walking in on that first day, and the guy was at the front, cooking with onions and garlic, and we had a whole lecture. If I remember right, he was speaking about the parasympathetic nervous system and parasympathetic responses to nutrition and how your satiety and hunger hormones are released just from the smell of the food. He's talking through it, and it just blew my mind! Immediately I can see links between nutrition and my performance and running.

After that first semester, I declared as a nutrition major with a minor in exercise science at Cornell University, and I ended up being a teaching assistant for then Prof. David Levitsky, who won all sorts of teaching awards; he's such a great instructor, and so I could stay and train with my buddies over the summer. I got a job as a lab tech in a vitamin E research lab that did vitamin E and cell culture and cancer research at the time.

I got into science then, but it still needed to be sports nutrition. After that time, I was excited, and I put applications in for chiropractic college and looked a little bit at med school. Still, that research experience ignited me in terms of my curiosity. I knew I wanted to return to Canada, as I was in the United States at that point, and I knew that the University of Guelph had good sports, nutrition, exercise science, and McMaster down the road. Guelph also had a good running programme, which I was interested in getting involved with in terms of coaching; I'm a level three international, middle-distance certified coach.

At that time, Lawrence Spriet was on sabbatical in Australia, working with Louise Burke and John Hawley. And it's the classic story – I don't remember you buying a used car just off the internet! You've got to see it; you've got to kick the tyres. Well, Lawrence had the same opinion or joke. This is pre-Zoom! We couldn't even talk! We talked on the phone once because it was a $40 phone call to Australia.

So Lawrence and I had some emails, and he sent me a big package of papers to read because you couldn't send attachments then. I heard later, behind the scenes, another legend in the sports nutrition field and caffeine research, Terry Graham, was also at Guelph.

I talked to Terry, as I used to race against his son, who was a good runner, but Terry's lab was full. Terry said, listen, Lawrence comes back from a sabbatical next year, he only has one or two students, and I think you'd be a great fit with Lawrence, but if he doesn't take you, I will. I guess Terry behind the scenes then called Lawrence and said, "Take Trent on", so I'm forever indebted to Terry for that!

So, the first time I met Lawrence, I would be a master's student. Lawrence is one of the biggest mentors I have. Lawrence and I started to do sports nutrition projects whilst I was coaching at the university and exercise science-type things, and just honestly, everything went from there. If I didn't get connected with Lawrence, I wouldn't be where I am today.

**It's fascinating to hear that, but it must be nice to reflect on it. This is the point; everyone starts somewhere, and there are always those "sliding door" moments in life I talked about a little bit in the first book, where you've almost got to jump, and the net will catch you, rather than deliberating or maybe not doing it.**

**Trent:** People say, oh, you know, you're so lucky. All these doors open for you. The people that the doors are opening for are pounding on 1000 doors. They're hustling. I contacted eight universities and 10 other professors when I returned from Cornell. I probably sent 20 applications/CVs out, but I only got about 10 replies. Yeah, and that's normal! So you have to hustle, you know.

So of the 10 replies, maybe eight agreed to meet with me – because they were lovely. Four were like, "My labs are full", so the stars lined up in the end. Still, there was a hustle behind there, too, to work through all these permutations and put a suit and tie on and come into an interview with a prof and the quasi interviews, but learn enough about their lab that I wasn't going to be ignorant walking in.

**It's crucial. Jill Leckey said she initially emailed Louise Burke from the UK to Australia and told me her Australian career would only have happened with that one email. So, another example of knocking on the door and speaking to the right people. You mentioned mentors and Lawrence in your early career. As you move through life and progress, sometimes those mentors change.**

**Trent:** The standout moment for me with Lawrence was the first American College of Sports Medicine meeting I attended, which is your equivalent of the European College of Sport Science (ECSS). I remember being with Lawrence, and he's so humble, so we're up early and walking to the conference, and he knows everyone, and I'm like, "We're gonna miss the talk!" And I was like, wow! So that impression upon me about his network and understanding a network and building a network and taking time to talk to people and be sociable and open and collaborative, and just a lovely person, imprinted upon me how to go through your career. Lawrence also helped set me up with a postdoc with Luc van Loon at Maastricht University. I was Luc's first postdoc, which was a great experience. My wife and I married and decided, "All right, we're moving to Europe!" So that was a bit scary, but we did it.

Then I got a job in Switzerland at Nestle with PowerBar, so we moved to Switzerland; again, challenging, but you have to go for it. So at Nestle, within PowerBar, we had excellent collaborative research set up with Louise Burke and John Hawley in Australia, Luc van Loon in the Netherlands, Stu Phillips in Canada, and Asker Jeukendrup in Birmingham at the time, and I was able to collaborate and get mentored for six or seven years by those individuals, whilst I was at Nestle. I was the primary project manager for PowerBar for the research and development, so I would go to those places, visit and help with the study designs, set them up and put enough work in to be a co-author on all those papers. That was a real galvanising time for being indirectly mentored by those people. It's important to state as well, and I may realise this more now than ever: at the Canadian Sport Institute, we have just unbelievable staff that I get mentored by every single day, and every level of the team, from grad students to interns and all those different relationships with staff and students, I'm a mentor to them, and they're a mentor to me. It's a great dynamic and a great environment to work in here.

**Just on PowerBar in Switzerland, were all of those links and networks already set up when you arrived, or is that something that you hit the ground running with?**

**Trent:** Great question. So, Nestle had just bought PowerBar, and they were setting up the sports nutrition piece within Nestle, and Nestle is a massive company, obviously £100 billion in sales and over 200 brands. There was a "Science Guy" in the business building, a guy named Eric Zaltas. Eric had been with PowerBar a long time, and I was the "Research Guy" in the research building. So Eric and I are still friends. We still text. Eric said he wanted to set up a bunch of research, and he asked me who did I think should be involved and what should we do?

I was in such an unbelievable position to say, if you want to do protein stuff, we have to talk to Luc and Stu, if you want to do carbohydrate, fuel and stuff, we're going to talk to Asker, and if we want to do training adaptation stuff, we're going to talk to John and Louise. So those relationships, especially the John and Louise relationship, as part of my PhD, featured a collaboration with them: the low carbohydrate availability/mechanism paper. That was my first paper with John and Louise!

I certainly knew those other people, but when you reach out, I'm not going to lie, it helps when you say, "Hey, we have some money to fund some studies!" So they answer their emails and engage quickly when you say stuff like that! We're all still great friends and colleagues, you know, it wasn't just about the money! I'm sure that smoothed the initial relationships when I kind of cold-called people and said, "Hey, we're in a position here to do some research."

PowerBar has now been sold, and they've gone a different way and no longer sponsor research. They're in a different situation now, but for those seven years, it was just full gas ahead and doing as many projects as we could.

**That's amazing, so with the move to Switzerland and PowerBar, those links might have been made as early on in your career and been as strong.**

**With your career now, is there a moment for you that stands out, whether that's an Olympic success or something you've achieved personally in nutrition? Do you have any standout moments?**

**Trent:** There are a couple; one is the very first time I got to go to significant games, working in sports science and nutrition. That was the 2006 Melbourne Commonwealth Games, a fantastic game with excellent facilities. My wife made that team; it was her first major game, and she made the final in the women's 1500m.

I had a few collaborative projects with Athletics Canada. They knew I was a sports nutrition/sports science guy, but again, I hustled and made a proposal via email to Athletics Canada. It was in the Melbourne Cricket Ground, and there were 100,000 people in that thing, and I was a postdoc at Maastricht University at the time, in Luc van Loon's laboratory.

I said, listen, this is March in Melbourne. It will be smoking hot, and you need some support for your athletes around fuelling. I see you have three race walkers, you have got three marathon runners, there are heat protocols, there are sports nutrition protocols. I said I had a place to stay. It was a combination of John and Louise's apartment in Melbourne, and a postdoc that used to be at Lawrence's laboratory, Matt Watt, who has his own publications in the *Nature* journal now.

I explained that I had a place to stay and would pay for my flight. I have my food and don't need to stay in the village. All I need is an accreditation.

I also explained that I could work with all these athletes. They agreed, and their response was, sure, okay. Funding my way as a postdoc (on a student's budget) cost us money at the time – but I wanted the opportunity! I already had relationships with some of these athletes.

But I was going anyway, and my wife was competing. I framed it so that it would be tough for them to say no!

This experience opened my eyes to all the pieces of performance and helping athletes. Then obviously, through my PhD, I knew John and Louise, and there's that sports science piece there. Then my wife made the final, and the weather was just perfect!

I turned 30, and my birthday was there. I remember they had a birthday party for me, and I was just like, I need to figure out how to do this full time. I knew that was such a galvanising moment where everything came together.

I had to go back to do a postdoc, as sports didn't employ me; I wasn't doing sports nutrition professionally. I was a postdoc at Luc's lab. That's what I would have to return to, but I knew that was where I wanted to go – it took 10 years to get there.

That was a standout, galvanising moment for me.

The second one was when we returned to Canada in 2011. A local, Canadian-broad philanthropy group called B2I0 (Business towards 2010), because we hosted the 2010 Vancouver Olympics, they contacted me as they have philanthropists who fund and do different sports projects in Canada. It's clean, and it's simple. They can see where their money's going. It's a lean organisation, but very high performance.

I was able to be a director and put together an applied two-year nutrition fellowship programme for applied sports nutritionists in Canada. About 20 people were involved, including mentoring and mentees and educational pieces, projects and professional development work. Six times over the two years, we all got together for three days in intensive workshops where we brought in people like James Morton, Louise Burke, Dave Martin, and Stu Phillips. I can go down the list. It was just a group of 20.

It was intensive; they would come in, and I've got pictures of Dave Martin with only about 10 of us telling stories until 2am about sport. That project was just so gratifying when I worked with the project on my return to Canada. That group is still tight. It spearheaded this entire rise of the quality of sports nutrition happening in Canada and the expectations around excellent service and innovative practice that's evidence based. That's one other substantial standout moment for me here in Canada.

**Did that happen once, or has that continued with a different cohort each year?**

**Trent:** No, it was a two-year programme with large legacy pieces that continue to happen with critical success factors, including how much are you contracted within the elite sport? How much did we shift that? We had one on endurance sport, and we had one on relative energy deficiencies in sport, we had one in sprinting, so there are a few different ways that they contribute back to the sport system, as well as working directly with certain athletes and teams to enhance what's going on in their environments. B210 has also run one for two years in mental performance, they've run just one-off workshops on a topic I helped organise, and now I consult with B210.

**Why do you think you, as an individual, have been so successful to date? And I appreciate that success can mean different things to different people, but why do you think you are where you are? What is it that you've done?**

**Trent:** So this is interesting! What do you mean by success? We must qualify this and consider it because do you mean successful as an applied sport scientist in the field working at the coalface? Or do you mean successful as a sports science researcher doing publications?

I want to hammer this home. Many people in the field, who are exceptional working in the area, feel they are only successful if they publish. I think that's a load of crap.

One of the best sports scientists in the world is Tim Kerrison. How many publications does that guy have? Still, you don't need to publish to feel successful working in the field. You can be highly successful and even more focused because doing research can be a distraction at some points. You need to be innovative; you need to be able to read the study and understand it enough to apply it, and you need to have a good network of researchers on your speed dial.

There's being successful as a human in society, being a good partner, being a good dad, taking time to volunteer, or being a good colleague at work. Being hyper-successful in one area can come at a cost in other areas. Can I get more publications? You bet. Am I sitting on datasets? Yep, but it will cost my family, my health and my relationship with my wife.

I can't do it anymore, even though I enjoy writing and working out datasets. I can't, so you come to grips with that and say, okay, I'll plug away on this, and you've got to learn to say no to specific pieces of your life to be successful.

Long story short, there's not one element.

I know this is going to be corny, but if I go back and I think about elements or what's an influential factor of success for me, I think it's going back to the first 18 years of my life and parents that instilled a good work ethic in me very early. My dad would sometimes have to go back to the shop to finish a job, or my mom was doing bookkeeping until 10pm, but they still volunteered at the church or were the assistant baseball coach, or all these other elements.

At the same time, you never take yourself too seriously. My dad is one of the funniest dudes you'll ever meet. He's got treatable prostate cancer, and the jokes he was telling at the hospital during COVID to go in and get a hormone shot... those traits, for me, are just so crucial to my success now.

Balancing those things, having some fun in life, and having a good laugh, you've got to grind. If you're not willing to work, it's not going to happen.

**What would you say has been the biggest challenge so far?**

**Trent:** This was a tough one, but I realised only a few years ago that not all professional working relationships can always work out. There are three or four professional relationships that I've had in my career that haven't worked out. It's not for lack of trying from me or them, and it's just for whatever reason, they didn't match.

It is still a dagger in my heart, like I have messed up. I remember talking to the guy who recruited me here. He passed away way too early from a heart attack: Dr Gord Sleivert. I struggled with one relationship when I first started here, and Gord was like, well, Trent, what's the divorce rate? I was 50%, he's like, yeah – we put such unbelievable expectations on our professional relationships; here's a partner that you've fallen in love with, you got a mortgage, you got kids, and you know, we've got to work at it.

I'm not telling you so that you think "There's another professional relationship lost and blown out the window!" It was just coming to grips with that a little bit. Yes, you always try to work at it. You try to be proactive and look at different personality styles and ways you work. Over my long career, three or four isn't too bad that just wouldn't quite jive, and we're able to figure out alternative solutions. Early in your career, no one tells you that! Like, hey, this might only sometimes work out.

You feel responsible and slightly guilty, like you're a bad practitioner. That was a challenge for me early on as someone who's quite goal oriented to come to grips with.

**On that, do you think back to the first, to the second, to the third, to the fourth instance, and do you think you've now managed to pick up on those signs where you feel this might not mesh between us?**

**Trent:** Yes. The most critical piece of that is expectation management. What is their expectation? And what is your expectation? If you need more clarity on that, that's when things will start to go sideways.

That can be as simple as working with a new coach and being proactive. How much, how often and in what style do you like to be communicated with? You're creating expectations around communication and feedback loops. I have some coaches that want to be attached to every single email to an athlete, I have other coaches where that upsets them, and they say quit filling up my inbox, do your job, let's meet for coffee once a month, and you'll bring me up to date on everything in between.

Let's talk about communication. Let's talk about availability. How often do you want to see me at the pitch versus not at the pitch? It's that expectation management, being purposeful upfront, and saying, "Hey, I'm new here; I want to work with you the best I can." You understand that I still do stuff for you behind the scenes when I'm not physically here.

**That's a significant bit of advice there. It's a huge one. I wish I had spoken to you sooner because I would have changed how I operated with an individual within my new place of work. We worked it out anyway, but that is the area that we could have done better at the beginning.**

**Trent:** Our task lists always need to be shorter. You are creating expectations about prioritising tasks that align with the person you're reporting to.

I always tell people to write down their tasks and send them to me. I go through and colour code: green, yellow and red. What do you think? Focus on the greens. If you have time for the yellows, let the reds sit. Let's have a look at this same spreadsheet in a month.

If I return to them and say, "Hey, why haven't you done this?" and they come back to me and say, "Well, you said it was red" then that's on me.

We're always prioritising, but we usually do that ourselves at our desks and need to sense-check it more. You can just have it, pull it out on paper at a coffee break with a coach. Just that simple process you're checking on a few times can also be beneficial because our task lists need to be shorter.

**To work in performance nutrition, what characteristics do you see in the people you look at that do very well in our industry?**

**Trent:** In a leadership course back at Nestle, we worked on a hierarchy piece with different permutations. Especially within sports nutrition, we are in a relationship-based discipline. The relationship pieces might not be as fundamental to your success as a biomechanist if you're good at math, methods and fundamentals of movements. You can find them online.

You can only succeed in sports nutrition with excellent soft skills! The same with mental performance. It's a relationship-built base.

At the base of this triangle, I would put personality traits, and then I would put values, then I would put relationships. Then at the top are education, skills, and experience.

## HIERARCHY OF TRAITS REQUIRED TO BE A WORLD-CLASS SPORTS SCIENCE PRACTITIONER

- EXPERIENCE
- SKILLS
- EDUCATION
- RELATIONSHIPS
- PERSONALITY

Figure redrawn with permission from Trent Stellingwerff

Everyone jumps in at education and skills and then tries to work towards experience without realising that the pyramid's base is your personality traits, values, and relationships. And we don't do a great job in most industries and fields at developing the bottom end of the pyramid and understanding how important that is.

There are whole areas of science on personality traits versus values. Values, nature, nurture, motivational interviewing, aspects of behavioural sciences and behaviour; we're in behaviour change.

Registered Dietitians will get a snippet of this stuff, but if you're coming in through university and more of an exercise scientist, I didn't have a single course on this in university. Not a single one. Just even the awareness that there are different personality styles. You can adjust your communication approach, and this can be key.

That's an area for sure, that bottom piece of the pyramid around personality, relationships, traits and values that are important to look at.

**It's a perfect point. How often do we see students gravitate through an undergraduate degree or a master's, and they get what you've just described? They're probably the top two or three layers of the pyramid, but you then put them in front of an athlete and ask them to talk or present, and they've yet to learn how to handle the situation.**

**If you've got the character and personality where you're okay in a room full of strangers, and you've got no problem going up and meeting people, you almost thrive in that environment because that's who you are. However, if you're different from that person and have the knowledge, some people need help.**

**I don't know of any courses in the UK in sports nutrition that teach you how to handle that situation or communicate and be a coach. Quite often in book 1, this area cropped up when I asked people the same question.**

**Trent:** Agree. I was a total nerd.

Do you have it in the UK, Toastmasters? There was a Toastmasters club. I only had time to make meetings, but it was impromptu communication, like boom, here's your topic. Go in front of everyone and talk. I did that in high school and then when I was at Nestle.

Communication, performance on demand, and of course that could be much fun for extroverts and just freakin' scary for introverts! But everyone would learn skills in that space to do a little better.

**What would be your biggest recommendation to your younger self or aspiring students entering the performance nutrition industry right now?**

**Trent:** Don't expect everything right away. Or even in 10 years; you need to be patient.

Unless you hustle, you'll probably be poor for a good time in the industry before you can make it.

If having enough money to feel secure is important to you, don't enter this industry! You can, through hustle, become comfortable in this industry, however. At our postdoctoral, Hillary (my wife) and I were on peanut butter and jelly for many years, which was a bit of a slog.

The second thing I would say is in that transition period, either from finishing university and maybe going into graduate school or a postdoctoral, or into your first couple of positions, perhaps those 10 years, if you want to excel in this industry, you have to be comfortable with having much change and taking some risks.

In that period between finishing my undergraduate degree, master's, PhD, and postdoc, and then coming here to Canada, that's a fifteen-year period where I lived in four countries. Six different advisors. Twelve different houses.

I am a homebody and more comfortable at home. My parents still live in the house I grew up in. We never moved once. Every one of those moves scared me. My wife is way more adventurous that way. She's like, we'll figure it out – let's go!

That's a piece you've got to come to grips with; developing a network, making those moves strategically, and taking some risk-taking will help your career in this space in the long run.

I'm nodding because you're describing where I am right now regarding that first eight-year period of your fifteen! As you're talking, I'm reflecting on my decisions over recent months.

Are there any things on courses in nutrition that we need to learn now that you think are essential? This comes back to that Toastmasters and behaviour side of stuff.

**Trent:** Behaviour management, motivational interviewing, and personality trait-type courses. In many methods, I'm going to age myself here. There has been a shift away from the hard biochemistry basics. You must slug it out with this stuff to understand metabolism, especially if you're innovative in sports nutrition.

More and more, the university courses are getting softer and softer in good old mechanistically based metabolism.

I came from a robust undergraduate in this area and then worked with Lawrence Spriet. I mean, that's his whole lab. He did his postdoc at the Karolinska Institute with Eric Hultman, who started the biopsy. That was hammered into us. This year, the International Sport and Exercise Nutrition Conference (ISENC) was a good example. Behind the scenes, Ron Maughan and I were messaging just on this topic. We said next year's ISENC, we want it to be very biochemistry based because he'd like the pendulum to swing back. In our opinion, as an industry, we have to nail these basics.

**I went through my studies at LJMU and fell into the trap of gaining lots of applied experience. However, there were numerous occasions when Graeme Close and James Morton would sit me down and say: read, get in the library and read, get the journals out, get the textbooks out and know the fundamentals because that is the underpinning of nutrition. I put my hand up and admit that I sometimes didn't do enough of that.**

**Where do you think nutrition will be in our industry in five years? There's much technology going on now, and there's a lot more data-driven stuff. Have you got any views on that?**

**Trent:** Yeah, a few of us did a session on this at the last ECSS, and out of it, we had a chance to write a mini-review in *Frontiers* that just got accepted on this topic. We've highlighted that in the 1990s, there were 50 sports nutrition papers a year, and last year, there were 3000. Yes, 3000. It's exciting times that there are 3000, but there's also absolutely no way there are 3000 good papers or good projects to publish. There aren't.

The amount of crap out there has exploded in combination with the explosion of the field. It's the explosion of journals and open-access journals where the review processes need to be more credible. That, coupled with the explosion of technology, of which the vast majority still needs to be validated technology, like what are there, 200 different downloadable apps for sleep on your phone right now? This means that it's going to become ever more critical to be able to see the signal from the noise. What is most important? What's validated? Which of these papers and studies are essential versus noise? It's exciting, but that's where we're going.

Sports nutrition, before 2000, was university-based exercise physiologists who were interested in nutrition who had the time to use validated equipment and make metabolic parts and work up the methods for muscle biopsies and measuring glycogen and muscle and assays – because if it wasn't validated, they couldn't publish, and so it wasn't worth doing.

Now, almost all your technology and new outputs are the exact opposite. They're not coming into the industry necessarily from a university point of view. They're coming out of it for profit, like a start-up business trying to balance a bottom line with its angel investor breathing down their neck who says they need a yield and return on investment in three to five years.

Therefore, they're willing to push the science for sales because if they don't, they're dead in three to five years anyway. Of course, it's an exciting time, but it's also a time when we need even more caution, common sense, and focus on the big rocks.

**Is there a book you've read recently that has improved your practice?**

**Trent:** I read every night for one hour outside of the field. A book I recently read that made me pause and think is *The Infinite Game* by Simon Sinek. He's got other good books like *Leaders Eat Last*. The book could have been 50% shorter because the best stuff, I think, is in the first three chapters, or 25% of the book. The rest of it is a regurgitation of that first 25%.

It's the idea behind a finite game. A game that ends and it's got rules, and it's got an ending, and it's got a winner, it's got a loser. It's like a football match. The infinite game is that you don't win or lose in life. You don't win at business. Even with death, hopefully, you have a legacy. Therefore, it has an infinite mindset, thinking, why am I doing this every single day? What are the relationships I have?

As you get older in your career and into your 70s, those relationships and those values mean the infinite game is much more critical than the finite game.

The juxtaposition of why this made me think is that all of our work in sports is where the outcomes are finite, but we need to take an infinite mindset into a limited environment. Because winning medals is how you get funding. I wouldn't say I like that because everyone's like, oh, it's all about the journey.

The journey is the infinite mindset. It's not about the outcome, the finite perspective. I'll reread the first 25% to refresh.

In the last couple of years, I have recommended that as something to pick up, think about, and ponder on yourself.

**I haven't read it, but I've listened to him on a podcast talk about this. It was something that James Morton and I had a chat about in our discussion, and it does make you sit and think about what you are trying to achieve. I can't help but think maybe that is also linked to the start of our conversation where you were talking about your two boys and you want to be at home,**

and you want to see the lads, and I wonder whether that has reframed a little bit of thinking there as well?

**Trent:** Yeah. Truthfully, I had come to discussions with my wife and others to shift my workload to be home more often before reading the book, and then the book came out, and it sat on the shelf for a year, and then I got through it, and it even further galvanised my decision.

**Are there any fundamental principles that you try and follow every day? So obviously, you mentioned there, an hour of reading every evening? Is there anything else that you try and keep in your daily life to keep Trent in sixth gear?**

**Trent:** My left knee has been an absolute killer since last summer. Personally, it has been rough lately. Until recently, I have tried running at least five days a week. I just saw an orthopaedic surgeon; I have a torn meniscus and am on the surgery list. Right now, I am training indoors on a bike versus outside. We have unbelievable trails 400 metres from our house; it is huge for us. The Olympic Rowing programme is 600 metres away. It has a beautiful lake. I've put on 12 pounds since stopping running and have probably eaten worse too. I am grumpy. I have gotten better at getting on the bike more often. In summary, I get some exercise every single day. My wife's now heading out for her run with a friend of hers. So yeah, exercise is a biggie.

**Finally, if you were to work with a performance nutritionist who you thought excelled at their role, what would make that individual who they are?**

**Trent:** I go back to my answer to the question about the characteristics. The framework I presented earlier about personality traits, values, relationships, and education skills and experience. That captures it well. Even within that triangle, the very peak of that triangle, they must have an innovative mindset. You can be experienced and good at your job, but you must be more clever. Note that I didn't use the word research. You can be world class without publishing research, but if you aren't creative and have an innovative mindset, that will set great practitioners apart from the good. An innovative perspective needs some level of strategic risk-taking within some group of the evidence base. Many people say they're creative, and it's just complete bullsh*t in terms of the evidence base. Also, you don't want to harm. Some level of risk-taking is okay. Risk-taking is required at the very top end of the sport for success.

**Considering everything we've discussed, the next person I interview could be Louise Burke. Is there a question that you would like to ask them?**

**Trent:** I would ask them that when they've lived a long, tremendous, industrious, and productive life, and they're 70 years old, they're 80 years old, what are their top two or three legacy pieces they want to leave behind? What are those in terms of their lives and contributions to our field if they could highlight some parts they feel proud of, like, boom, we moved the needle on this, and everyone practises differently?

**It's been amazing to chat, and I appreciate your time.**

**Trent:** Keep up the great work. Please consider opening your scope and including everything I said here – it would work in any discipline, in all sports science.

## JAMES'S THOUGHTS

Trent is one of the world's best applied researchers in sport nutrition. What I love about this interview is how honest and open he was regarding the early days, from receiving packages of papers to read from Lawrence Spriet in the post due to email attachments not being a thing, to hustling as a young student contacting universities for interviews.

How many people hustle like that in today's world?

Trent has done some serious air miles too, from Switzerland to Australia for the Commonwealth Games, and of course to and from Canada, his home. He also explains how it isn't all about publishing papers; you can be a great applied researcher without the need to publish your work.

Finally, there is a gem of advice in this chapter regarding communication with people you work with. Read that section again as it is gold and one that reminds me of so many of my own situations in sport.

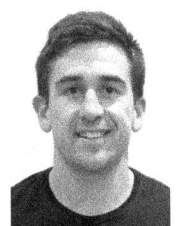

## CHAPTER 2:
# DR DAVID DUNNE

David completed his PhD at Liverpool John Moores University in digital health and behaviour change. He is the owner of Hexis, a new technology which provides personalised nutrition powered by AI. He consults to the Ryder Cup golf team and has previously worked as a performance nutritionist with Harlequins Rugby and Olympic sports.

David and I first met at the International Sport and Exercise Nutrition Conference in Newcastle around eight to nine years ago. It was evident from our first meeting that not only did we both enjoy a beer, but we were both enthusiastic and passionate in coaching athletes in performance nutrition strategies.

David at the time was working with Harlequins Rugby and I was just about to start my master's in sports physiology, so it was great to meet him at this pivotal point in my own career.

We have since stayed in touch, become great friends, and continually support one another with business ideas, applied projects and career paths.

You can follow David on:
Twitter @david_m_dunne
Instagram @david_m_dunne, @hexis.live, @hexis.recipes

**The first part of this is an introduction to yourself. Who are you, and what is your background? How have you gone from studying and working in sports to what you're doing now?**

**David:** I'm David Dunne. My background is in performance nutrition, where I've worked for the last 10-plus years as an applied practitioner across various sports. I started in professional rugby, football and fencing simultaneously, so I was fortunate to get exposure to different sports with unique challenges, especially fencing, as I had no background. This made me realise the value of being exposed early in your career to something you've never seen. So that spurred me on to get involved in quite a few more sports. I was always interested from a practitioner's side in what I could do to evolve and develop my applied skill set. That led me back towards academia, where I self-funded a PhD in behavioural design thinking and technology innovation in applied sports nutrition. Where I am right now, I am entering my second career. I recently co-founded a start-up called Hexis, where I and a team of PhDs are currently building a sports technology platform to help people fuel their training demands.

**You were one of the people doing a substantial amount of nutrition support. How have you found that transition from being the practitioner on the ground to not too much now?**

**David:** I found it challenging but enjoyable because there's been much growth. I've been exposed to many things that I've never been exposed to before. As a result, I've had many more opportunities to learn by stepping outside the discipline of nutrition and the sports field and entering the world of business, finance, and technology.

From a personal perspective, it rounded me a bit more as a person in the world when my prior experience in sports kept me in an echo chamber. It has been challenging as well. You enter another planet, and you're a complete novice. I still have lots to learn, but I enjoy the experience. I would also say on that side of things, meeting different people who are trying to solve the same problem but approaching it from a completely different angle has been fascinating and broadened my perspective as to what can be done when we get a genuinely multidisciplinary team in a room and working together.

**How and when did you first get involved in nutrition? What was your first experience of actual nutrition delivery and exposure?**

**David:** I was fortunate that I was interested in it from a very young age. Nutrition and sports science have interested me quite heavily since about 13. So right away, throughout secondary school, I picked my subjects and worked my schoolwork around, knowing I wanted to get into strength and conditioning or nutrition. I managed to get a couple of placements in both disciplines. I realised I had a bigger passion for nutrition because I liked the variety and got involved in service delivery towards the end of my undergraduate degree. I was able to take up a role at Bradford Bulls professional rugby league club when they were in the Super League. It was a great experience because I was only 21 and essentially presented to and helped prepare a first-team senior squad. I learned more from them than they learned from me, but that's all part of the process.

**Throughout your career, you've been one who has not been afraid to travel for your jobs. So then, you would have been in London, but you were travelling up to Bradford?**

**David:** Yeah, a seven-hour mega coach. I would travel up on a Sunday night by coach to get there on Monday, then do a couple of days up there, and then travel back. Budgets were tight at the time, and even the train was off limits. I've always thought you can't say no if there's an opportunity. You must figure out a way to make it work. The whole time I was based in London, working across various sports. Because I got off to that start where you must travel for the opportunity, you must make it work on your side, not theirs. That became the norm. Some options were London based, but many weren't UK based, and that's part of the nature of this game, just rolling with it. It might also be one of the problems. It's probably why we see some practitioners transitioning in their 30s, like myself, into their second career or pivoting. There's potentially a sustainability issue when we're looking at the lifespan of an applied practitioner.

I know I've had a couple of years where I spent between 50 and 100 days a year on the road, which, compared to what other people do on the World Tour cycling, it's nothing. But at different life stages, you have different priorities and opportunities. So, it's interesting, and I keep a keen eye on it. I am always fascinated to hear people's stories and journeys because I wonder, are some aspects of the applied practitioner role a younger person's game?

**I know many practitioners working in motorsport and Formula One. The race calendar requires much travel, and at what age do you accept that that will be your whole life and what you would have done your entire career?**

**David:** For some people, that's exactly what they want to do. Fair play; it might only be for some. As you said, Formula One is a good example where you're looking at 200-plus days a year on the road. You've got to love it, you've got to live it, you've got to breathe it, you are part of it, your identity is tied to it, and for some people, that's exactly what they want. For others, it's not. It's completely okay. Either way, everyone must find what works for them, even if it's okay for some time, and then it stops being okay or the other way around. Then that's part of everyone's chapter to their life, I suppose.

**So, in terms of mentors, for you and your career, who would be a standout person or persons and why?**

**David:** I had one mentor from my early days as a practitioner. I was fortunate to be part of a good sports science and medicine department at British Canoeing (BC). I also worked on the canoe sprint programme and moved to the slalom programme. But when I started on the sprint programme, our head of performance was Dr Brian Cunniffe. Brian is a performance scientist, and he's done much previous work. Part of his PhD might have been in nutrition as well. But he wasn't a practising nutritionist at BC. He was a performance scientist and the head of performance. But he would be a standout person that's helped shape me, and my thought process over the years. He never gave me any answers. You'd always be in a meeting with Brian, and he would ask the questions that would get you thinking in the right direction and would help you figure out how to progress things with your team or yourself or the athletes that you're working with or the problems that you're looking to solve. One of the most significant roles he's played has been around critical thinking and trying to bring that out, and I'm very grateful to him for that. I still work with Brian to this day, and I'm always keen to work with him on any projects because he's got a unique skill set which I don't think should ever be taken for granted. I'm very grateful to have that, and he keeps asking me those questions to this day that keep the cogs turning in the right direction as well.

**What's been a standout moment for you in your career?**

**David**: This is an interesting one because there have been lots of highs and lows. Everyone's involved in lots of highs and lows, and most practitioners that have been involved in sports for a period have been lucky enough to experience some level of success, whether in the Olympics or it's in professional sports. I've been fortunate enough to be involved in several Olympic medals, world titles and golf Ryder Cups. But a standout moment for me is in the family. My brother is a professional golfer. I think seeing his development through university, coming into the elite game, post college, and making his debut at the Golf Open was probably one of those standout moments. It was his second Open then, and seeing him leading after 72 holes was remarkable. To sit and be part of and watch someone close to you deliver on that stage was incredible. He's been progressing since then, and he'll carry on moving. But those moments supporting my family in the elite world of sports are the ones I hold closest.

**How did the Open end for your brother?**

**David:** He didn't have the best Sunday (final day of competition) but had a fantastic competition. He missed out on a silver medal; a silver medal at the Open is essentially the highest-placed amateur. It was an experience, and he took a lot from it. The whole family was there watching, and I don't believe many things compared to that. The only thing I could compare it with was when he won the British Masters a few years later. I'm sure he'll have a few more chances soon, and I'll make sure I'm there for them.

**When I ask this question about being successful, that can be any way you define success because some people would look at Michael Jordan and say he's the successful one, but others would look at getting a degree and say they were successful. What do you think has been the most influential factor as to why you've succeeded in your early career?**

**David:** It's a good question. It's all relative, like you said, from a success perspective. In many ways, it's subjective in terms of what success is. There are a couple of things. As I said at the start, getting exposed to a range of sports I had no background in or knowledge of helped me early on.

I understand how to problem solve and figure things out, working with coaches and finding ways to have impacts when I need to become more familiar. It's also humbling; you're a novice in some environments. You still need to help find ways to help those athletes. I got my first role in professional sports in 2012. Getting exposed to a wide range of sports early on has helped me personally. Also, putting people first, putting people ahead of athletes, and recognising humans ahead of statistics and numbers has helped me build relationships with people. If I bumped into them today, I'd still be very comfortable sitting down, going for lunch, and having a good catch-up. But investing in people and relationships has helped. That's how I approach situations anyway. I'm fascinated by people and different people's stories, why they think the way they think and what they want to do, and how I could help them realise their potential or even listen sometimes. I believe building relationships probably comes out on top there.

**What's been the biggest challenge of your career to date?**

**David:** I have a standout moment on this, which probably led to my career change. I remember being at Harlequins Rugby back in 2014. I remember sitting down with a player and the player saying, just looking at me, I know what I need to do. I'm sitting here in front of you. His attitude was, you can tell me something I don't know, but at the end of the day, I just don't want to do it. In the role, you do everything you can to help everyone, educate, and ensure the kitchen is how it should be and that the service delivery team has the necessary resources.

That was a humbling experience for me. This player was an unbelievable character and still is. He knew what to do, why he should do it, and the negative consequences of not doing it, but ultimately, he wasn't motivated to do it. That was the experience that led me to want to explore the behaviour side a little bit more because, at the same time, I had started to self-fund a PhD looking at social media. Social media was the bit that was influencing people. But I began to realise that it wasn't social media. Technology is a medium, and we must help people change their behaviour. That was probably one of my biggest career challenges, realising I was not qualified to do what I needed to do with this person. Because I needed to understand how to influence his behaviour, alter his motivation levels and change his thought process around these scenarios to be impactful.

You go through a university system at that stage and acquire knowledge and information. You enter different environments, and people speak about soft skills and building relationships. And yes, you can build relationships. You can build trust. But you must teach yourself at university how to deliver behavioural interventions or work with people displaying these characteristics. That was a challenge and probably motivated me to look at this more. On a personal level, I never actually really thought I wanted to do a PhD because I looked at a lot of the heavy molecular side, and I was like, look, I like to learn about this. But I can't get this deep into it for the next three or six years. But when it came to people, I wanted to learn more. That was probably the biggest challenge. But also, it's created quite a lot of opportunities as well.

**With your experience and the number of nutritionists you have worked with, had as interns or via work experience, what are the characteristics you see in those people that you believe people need to work in nutrition?**

**David:** This is a good question. Everyone's individual, so I don't want this to come across to people as if they don't have these things, then they shouldn't be working in nutrition because who am I to say what's right? I could be completely wrong, and I have my own bias, so I'm anchored in a specific direction. Regarding applied nutrition and working in a professional setting with athletes, particular characteristics can lend themselves to team and individual sports. A couple of things that come out quite consistently are people that can build relatedness with other people, so the ability to relay empathy, to be compassionate, and to listen. There are three essential things. One, the ability to think critically about a situation, two break down the different variables, and three understand where nutrition sits in this puzzle. I'd have everything here. That's, let's say, trying to make the boat go faster. You know, how important is this? And how important is this right now? The last thing I would say is being inquisitive.

From my perspective, I am sitting here with my bias. Some practitioners are naturally inquisitive and willing to spend time learning more, not because they feel they need to know more but because there's a genuine interest in wanting to help someone and trying to figure this kind of thing out. But if I were to put that inquisitiveness, coupled with intrinsic motivation, the ability to be empathetic, compassionate, and listen critically, that will be a nice bundle.

**If you were to enter the industry now with everything you know, what would be your recommendations to David Dunne at 18 or aspiring students trying to break into nutrition?**

**David:** I would recommend people figure out their super strength early, and get exposed to those different environments, so you can understand what you are good at – what would separate you from everyone else in your class? Because so many practitioners are coming out now, that having this base level of knowledge and ability to execute is a given, but everyone should have that. But I would always ask, what makes you different? What makes you unique? Why do I give you this job over the 25 people that sit beside you? I look at even our peer group and see how different people have become experts at other things. When hiring certain people and people being pulled into specific roles, many people are drawn in because of something they're good at, knowing they have a decent level of everything else. But again, I could be wrong. There's nothing to say I am right. But that would be my advice if somebody was coming out now. If somebody is worried that they're not this good at this but exceptional at something else, get excellent at what you're good at and get the other bit to an acceptable level. You can continually improve. But something is going to need to separate you.

**I presented recently at a conference in Nottingham, and I asked how many in the audience had a vision. Where is it they want to get to? Three people put their hands up. Two were staff, and one was a student. Some of them were saying, at this age now, I am still determining where I want to be. It's easier to figure out if you get the exposure and sit down and think about it like I could now. One of my super strengths is building rapport and relationships and getting people to buy in to something.**

**David:** You hit the nail on the head. It must come with exposure. I was lucky that during my undergraduate, I actively sought out any role to help any team for any period to get some experience. Many people wait till after their undergraduate to get some experience. Suppose people can frontload that a bit more and get those answers quicker. Then maybe they get some background on a master's, and then suddenly, that's another few years before you can generate revenue and get paid for what you do. Something which took me a long time to figure out, and I wish I'd seen these kinds of things when I was a bit younger, is to start with your why. What is your why? I think that identifying that even at 18, I don't necessarily believe that core why changes – your ability to articulate what it is probably improves.

If I look back now, in terms of why I've done something, I have always done it for one reason and one reason only and to this day, it still is – and I've probably just repurposed from being in the applied side to being in the technology side to try to do it at scale now – I love to do what I do to help people realise their potential. I love that whole area, whether it's my brother or someone else, that concept of potential for somebody, and not on a selfish level being part of that, but just being able to see somebody develop. That led me down the behaviour route, leading me to more of the human way. That's probably why everything stemmed off the back of that. For me personally; for somebody else, it could be something else.

**When studying at university, were there areas you didn't learn? Modules that you think would have benefited you as a practitioner?**

**David:** When I did my undergraduate, I did a joint honour. I majored in nutrition, did a minor in sports science at St. Mary's University of London and had a great time. But sports nutrition was a module in the third year. And then, after that, I did a postgraduate diploma from the International Olympic Committee during its early years. I was part of the first few cohorts where the course was still developing. There was lots of stuff that needed to be covered, and there was lots of stuff that was covered, maybe in less detail as we know now because the research has evolved. And all those courses have significantly improved as the volume of research and our understanding of biochemistry, exercise physiology and physical performance improved. I would love to have understood behaviour a little bit more. I would have loved to have been taught more about working with people. That comes down to some people being better than others anyway; some people like yourself have a more innate ability to build a relationship based on your personality. But I would have loved to have learned about that. I would have also loved to have known more about dietary periodisation, although it's a recent advancement in the field. Many people like John Bartlett, James Morton and Sam Impey are pushing that on. I've always liked the nuance in that area, I have to say, but those two areas probably, I would have enjoyed.

If the world was the way it is now, technology would be something I'd also be interested in. I still play sports, and I got into training, and I'm one of the old guys in the team. I hear the 19/20-year-olds at college talking about how they're learning about different Amazon Web Service platforms and how it all connects. When I was at university, we were sitting on Facebook, and people were getting into Instagram. If you wanted to know what happened Wednesday night, people were tagged in pictures on Thursday morning. Different ballgame, but that's just the rate and pace of change. So now that will be interesting to learn about because it's so prominent in our lives, but it wasn't even relevant at university.

**Where do you think the future of nutrition will be in five years?**

**David:** Nutrition is at an exciting crossroads at the minute, where the future of food will become a lot more personalised than what it is. In the physical performance space, we're seeing the evolution of tools, like the Oura Ring, Whoop and all these different wearable devices that continuously capture a range of physiological variables.

I can see personalisation and periodisation coming into it. Hopefully, Hexis and what we're working on will be a big part of that.

We will start to understand a lot more about genetic profiling. We've seen some stuff around caffeine already and fast and slow responders, those kinds of things. There's a lot more for us to learn there. The absolute cusp of it will be this hybrid approach; there will likely be a stage where humans and technology work together instead of just humans. There will likely be scalable and continuous tech-enabled solutions that will help people daily, anchored around the human helping them.

**Is there a book you've recently read that has improved your practice? It doesn't necessarily have to be nutrition based.**

**David:** There are two books. The first book is a book called *Zero to One* by Peter Thiel. It's more of an entrepreneurial book, but looking at how you may have a contrarian belief and that's okay. Maybe it's because you see something different. Perhaps because you're seeing something different to everyone else, you may have an insight that others don't have at that stage. I encourage people to read that book if they're interested in business. It's applicable, and if you're trying to run your own business as well, it's good to challenge some of our thought processes as it speaks about horizontal versus vertical progress. The idea of going from zero to one means it still needs to be done, and then you do something. So, there's some vertical progress there, you've gone from zero to one, as opposed to more horizontal progress where somebody has done something and maybe they've done it 10 times, and now you go from 10 to 11.

The other one would be, as you mentioned, Simon Sinek, *The Infinite Game*, bringing to life some of the work of Professor James Carson. What I like about that is how it positions us in this world of performance, nutrition, or sports, whatever way we want to look at it. That no one wins it, no one loses. Yes, people win competitions in a year. But over the course of your career, you join the game, you are a player in that game for some time, and the game's rules will change. You could change one of those rules. You could introduce a new way to play the game; that fascinates me, finding a new way to play the game.

But at some point, you will leave, and new players will come in, and this will continually evolve. It'll be here long after we pass. In terms of framing things, I also liked that book. And it's a pretty friendly reminder that we're all working towards the same goal, really, and it's, in many ways, how can we help each other in this game because our job is to help others anyway. But collectively and collaboratively will be better than just looking at that individually.

**I've listened to a lot of his stuff. Susie Ma, on the High-Performance podcast, also mentions *The Infinite Game*. She introduces it to Jake Humphrey and Damian Hughes because they have yet to hear it and have a fascinating discussion.**

**Are there any fundamental principles you try to follow every day now that you have left London and returned to your homeland, Ireland? Are there key things that David Dunne does to remain David Dunne?**

**David:** Good question. I need to improve on this is the honest answer with an open book. I struggle more with the work-life balance. It may tilt more in the work direction because it fascinates me. It's more of a hobby. Some days it's a job, and some days, it feels like a job. But most days, it feels more like a hobby. Instead of every day, I think: look, ensuring I get some form of physical activity throughout the week is essential. If that starts to go, I begin to lose my mind a bit. Self-care and the ability to practise what you preach is probably one of those.

**In your eyes, what makes a successful performance nutritionist in our industry?**

**David:** It depends on the organisation, their needs, and the practitioner's job for that specific place. But I'd return to what I said earlier about some essential characteristics. I think somebody that can show empathy, be compassionate, and listen to ultimately build that relationship and relatedness, can problem solve through critical thinking and has a decent level of intrinsic motivation to be able to figure things out, even if they don't know it – I think are all important. There needs to be a fundamental level of knowledge and understanding of biochemistry, exercise physiology, how the body works, and how it responds to food and different scenarios. I will take it that that is a given that we should all have. But they're the bits I'd layer on top.

**And then just a final one from me. This book is all about understanding the navigation of how practitioners like yourself, like me, like Trent Stellingwerff and Louise Burke, have worked our way through our careers. Are there any other thoughts or anything else you want to add that might help or support those who are either beginning their career or are stuck at a crossroads?**

**David:** I think the one thing I'd say, which is standing out now, is being a bit agnostic towards opportunities: don't feel like because you didn't get a job in a sports team, you don't want to take a position in another place. The field of performance nutrition and sports nutrition is evolving rapidly. In five years, there will likely be jobs that aren't currently available, that could be more centred around innovation, that could be more centred around an area that exploded, so don't get too narrow too soon.

In the next 10 years, as I said, there will be a whole range of new jobs that don't even exist at the moment. They don't even have a title that you will probably have a skill set for and be well suited to, so remaining a little bit open on that side of things is perhaps one thing I would say.

## JAMES'S THOUGHTS

What I love about David's interview is the way he openly talks about the career pivots he has made along his journey, from Bradford Rugby, to Harlequins, to now running a business to do with artificial intelligence and technology.

One area that stands out is the part about when the athlete knows what to do, but just doesn't want to do it. I have been in these situations before and I often reflect back on what I could have done differently to get the athlete to "want" to do it. Was my approach wrong, was the carrot I dangled wrong or not enticing enough? I think the practitioners who can get the buy-in, and get athletes to want to do it, are the ones who get great outcomes.

David's advice on you, the reader, knowing your super strength early on is also a gem. We are all different; we all have our own unique twist which makes us who we are. Reflect on what yours might be, embrace it, double down on it and use it to your advantage.

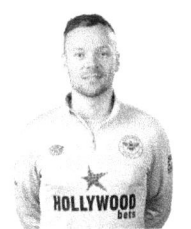

# CHAPTER 3:
# TED MUNSON

Ted is currently the performance nutritionist with Premier League team Brentford Football Club, having helped them with promotion last season. He also runs his own consultancy company where notably he consults to a multi-championship Formula One team.

I first met Ted when he worked at Science in Sport as a performance nutritionist. Professor James Morton spoke highly of Ted, and it was evident from when I first met him how driven he was, not only for his own training but also in his strategies for the athletes he works with.

We have often spoken on the phone in the car regarding our own careers, how we can learn from one another and also areas we think are going to be helpful in the near future in the field of nutrition.

Ted is a keen runner, having done many endurance events including trail runs. He often shares insightful content on his social media platforms which are a must to follow if you are a student keen to learn off a leading nutritionist in sport.

You can follow Ted on:
Twitter @TedMunson
Instagram @tedmunson.nutrition

**First question: who are you, and what is your background?**

**Ted:** I'm Ted Munson. I've been a sport and exercise nutritionist (registered) for five years. I've been involved in elite sports since I finished my BSc in 2014.

When I went to university in 2011, I didn't know what I wanted to do. All I knew was that I wanted to work in sports with professional athletes in some capacity, whether that be strength and conditioning, fitness, coaching, performance analysis etc.

I studied sports coaching and science at the University of Hull because I was into tennis and football coaching then. That could be a career path for me, especially if working with elite athletes was too far away. In my final year of studies (2014), there was an opportunity from Hull City Football Club. The club was looking for a first-team sports science intern. A small group of students, including myself, were offered to interview, and that was the first time I thought working in elite sports could be an option.

Six of us were chosen to interview for this sports science internship role, and at the time, I thought I didn't have any chance of getting it. I remember thinking that even the sports psychology lecturer who put us all forward was quite sour about my options. Some of the other students I was up against had been professional rugby league players previously, and another had experience working with elite athletes in an analysis role. I remember thinking: I'm not sure how I will get this! In the interview, I will go for it and display my knowledge and personality. I ended up getting the role.

I remember asking the head of performance, Will Royal, why he chose me over these students with much more experience. Will said the other guys might have been professional sportspeople with more experience, but you would fit better in this environment with this manager.

I never thought of that at the time. I'd never even thought about the environment and culture. They found me a little less serious, but I still had the knowledge to back up my point when needed. There may be different environments where that kind of relaxed attitude might not work, but in this case, it was what Will was looking for as a junior practitioner.

Based on this experience and many other interviews since then, it's hard to give that immediate advice on landing that first role. How you should be is subjective; perhaps if the head of performance had a different philosophy, I wouldn't have landed that role. Other managers, performance directors, etc., set different environments, and one practitioner might not fit into another domain. That's why it's essential to adapt to different environments but always stick to your core values as a practitioner.

I got that first opportunity at Hull City and was straight in at the deep end! One other sports scientist left to join another club soon after I joined. The new lead sports scientist I reported to also worked with England football then. I remember there were times he was away with England, and I was the only sports scientist at the Premier League club, analysing the GPS, hydration testing, body weights, making up all the protein shakes, preparing for games etc. It was incredible! I was well and truly embedded in the club. I didn't even attend my graduation ceremony because I was on a plane to Portugal for pre-season training.

I was thrown in at the deep end, and it was hard. I learned so much, made many mistakes and had lots of success. That's how I got into elite sports.

Now in terms of nutrition, being a Premier League club, in 2014 they had a nutritionist called Shane Thurlow who was in the club twice per month. I keep in touch with Shane today and published a hydration paper with him two years ago. He's a great researcher based out of Leeds Beckett University. Shane would come in, and I would pick up many things from him regarding what to give the players. Essentially, I would deliver what Shane was directing, and that's when I saw the benefits nutrition had on performance. I also saw the gap where some players needed to focus on nutrition. It was clear that there was an opportunity for me to specialise in performance nutrition and make a real impact.

This was about halfway through my first year of the internship, and I was in the process of starting a master's in research at the University of Hull alongside my internship. I was going to do it on GPS and strength and conditioning, but I found nutrition interesting. At the time, Hull University didn't have a nutrition department; now, they do, and it's registered with the British Dietetics Association.

I wanted to do a hydration study with the Hull City Football Club players, but collecting the data I needed "in season" was challenging. I also worked with some elite tennis players, so I decided to base my study around them. Although I was doing a master's in nutrition as a topic, it was officially a master's in sport and exercise science. When I finished that master's, I couldn't then technically be a Registered Nutritionist, although I was doing nutrition-related work, day in and day out, at Hull City.

This kind of practice was "allowed" at the time. I know many people were doing that, and in my eyes at the time, I thought, well, I've done a master's in nutrition, hydration, and working in it on a day-to-day basis, but obviously, I still needed to get accredited. That's when I researched the Sport and Exercise Nutrition Register (SENR). I then completed a postgraduate diploma in sport and exercise nutrition with Leeds Beckett University, which gave me the credits to join SENR. During this time, I left my role at Hull City to take up the part of performance nutritionist at Science in Sport (SiS), the supplement company. At the time, that role was focused on supporting their sponsored elite athletes. They helped Team Sky, USA Cycling and countless football teams, and I saw it as a good opportunity but very different from the "team sport" environment. I saw it as an opportunity to work with many other athletes.

I didn't know it would put me in touch with different people in the industry, including yourself [James]. People like David Dunne and James Morton I might not have met as early as I did. SiS gave me the platform there and allowed me to demonstrate my ability as a practitioner to numerous people. I was at SiS for three years and decided to leave in early 2019. My role at SiS changed a lot; it became corporate for me, and it was clear that I wanted to be back into the day-to-day sports performance environment.

I developed as a practitioner during my time there. I had the opportunity to see a lot of different environments, go into many other clubs and various sports, like cycling, and get a whole rounded approach. That helped me develop my philosophy, which we'll go into shortly.

I set up my own company four years ago; this is the best thing I did for my career. Leaving the comfort of full-time employment was risky, but I'd made many contacts. I started with a role at Millwall Football Club one day a week alongside a supplement development role at a company called Blue Fuel, which at the time partnered with Chelsea Football Club. Shortly after starting this, I secured a contract with Birmingham City Football Club, supporting for one day per week. As my days began filling up, I also marketed performance nutrition services for endurance athletes, which I am keenly interested in. I started my own company and had contracts with two championship clubs. I remember struggling with organising the days of support as they would often conflict. I still struggle with that now. I remember trying to fit a complete squad body composition analysis, six individual 1-1s, two staff meetings and a performance restaurant planning session into one day – not recommended! You've got to be organised and deliver what you can; don't spread yourself too thin.

In mid-2019, I made a big step and started a role with the Harlequins Rugby Union team in London. It was a real challenge because I needed to learn more about rugby union then. I learned much about the physical side of things but needed more about the game's rules and details. This role was a step out of my comfort zone. I started the job three days per week at Harlequins alongside Millwall and Birmingham City FC. Things changed because of COVID-19, and Millwall didn't have the budget after COVID-19 to keep my role going, so that stopped.

I found myself in a hole during COVID-19. I think everybody did. As a contractor, it made my role high risk and yeah, I lost positions because of it. I reflected. First, I needed to use that time to develop as a practitioner. After some time, I got myself into a better place where I was reading more and developing. I read about sports nutrition, like psychology and behaviour change. I also used that time to build my business as well. I worked with four or five international endurance athletes, some of whom I still support today.

When COVID-19 finished, I was lucky to see my career further accelerate. Two years ago, I joined Luton Town Football Club. In early 2022 I started supporting a Formula One (F1) team. I relished this opportunity being a big F1 fan and since F1 is relatively unresearched from a sports science perspective. This role involves working with the travelling support staff, which has thrown many challenges my way and, more importantly, the opportunity to find solutions to human performance. If you can look after the team that powers the car, you can see real gains in performance on the track.

At the end of the 22/23 season, I left Harlequins Rugby to join Brentford Football Club. This role is three days a week and allowed me to work alongside my other jobs with a developing team in the Premier League.

To summarise, I work with Brentford Football Club, Luton Town Football Club and an F1 team.

**What was your first involvement in nutrition?**

**Ted:** It was at Hull City when I was meeting with Shane Thurlow every month, and he was guiding me on how to set the players up with individualised protein shakes, and performing hydration testing, then feeding that data back to the players, so that would be my first "This is performance nutrition" role. There was also the admin side of things which can come as a surprise to new graduates. Things like supplement ordering, collecting and storing the batch tested certificates, general physiological data collection etc. That was my first involvement.

**Who are some of the most significant mentors in your life, and why have they been essential for you too?**

**Ted:** Firstly, a recent mentor is to do with my business. I was raised in a family that all worked in the public sector. No one knew about a company, how to set up a company, how to deal with accounts and how to potentially grow that company. My mentor also had a start-up company a while ago, and it has developed into a sports coaching business and a separate property development company. I recommend anyone looking to start their own company to seek advice from people that have done it before!

In terms of nutrition, I need help to pick one person out. I had to think about this; who is someone, that one person with whom I can have deep conversations, and I probably don't have that? That might be surprising, but I don't have just one individual.

There are certainly a few people I know that I could call upon anytime and have done a lot more in the past compared to now. I class people like David Dunne as someone I could call and chat with anytime, and I have done so in the past. Andy Kasper, I did some work with him in the past and knew I could call him anytime. Even more recently, I set up some work with Nessan Costello. He is on my wavelength. Indeed, that's something that I need to do, increase my support system in performance nutrition. Students should do this as soon as possible, and I will follow my advice here! Find someone who's been there, done it, made the mistakes, and is much better than you.

I enjoy spending time with people in our area, but finding mentors nowadays is challenging because people are challenged for time. I'm mentoring three students – we have calls every two weeks or so, and they're constantly messaging me and asking for advice. We keep it informal, grab a coffee and run through ideas, challenges, and solutions. I end up taking more away than they think. Two have landed roles as performance nutritionists, and the other isn't far off. Building a network to learn and demonstrate what you can do is essential. Many nutrition roles nowadays come through word of mouth.

I do have performance coach mentors. For years, I've worked with a fitness coach called Sean Rush. I have followed him around since he was at Leeds United back in 2016; even in 2011, he was at Hull City when we first started talking. Sean is now at Birmingham City Football Club, where I've consulted for the last few years. I go to him for anything on the performance side, whether GPS, fitness, or anything like that, because he's seen everything, made mistakes, and had plenty of success. He's probably dealt with well over 10 managers in his time. Sean is one of those people I always ask for advice.

In summary: build mentors of varying different levels of seniority. Look outside nutrition and those who work in sports science. Multidisciplinary learning is critical! Bounce ideas with people like you, create practitioner WhatsApp groups and share ideas.

**What's been a standout moment in your career to date?**

**Ted:** The first thing I think of is the first time you win something as a team or with a particular athlete. It is the biggest standout because you're ingrained in the group. You see the ups and downs and go through a year supporting them, and then everything comes together when they lift that trophy. That is it for me.

You ask your partner, and she says you're constantly watching the games on TV at the weekend. It consumes your life. When I was at Harlequins Rugby, it was huge when they won the Premiership title in 2021, and that was the first time I'd ever won something significant. It was my second season with the team. We finished sixth the year before. Something happened that year. We had a managerial change, we ended up having no head coach, and the other coaches stepped up, increasing player involvement.

I reflect on that time in my life and think about what went right there for us to do that. I certainly think about my situation. What went right for me? What did I implement to facilitate that winning performance? That was a standout moment for my career because that taught me about a few things, like self-reflection.

As a student, you believe self-reflection is just that annoying thing at the end of each module that you must do, but the learnings from that season have positively influenced the last two years of my career. I think about that all the time. I reflect on previous learnings and implement certain practices based on those learnings. I think about the environment and the culture that season, and little things like changes in the meals, bringing the players' involvement into the menu planning, and certainly putting the player as a person first and an athlete second. As a practitioner in a team, it's not all plain sailing, and I wouldn't change those ups and downs at all.

**What do you think has been the most influential factor as to why you've been successful today? What is it that Ted's got that allows Ted to get the roles, stay in the positions and do a good job?**

**Ted:** It's how I fit into an environment. I'm not overly serious and try to strike that "banter vs serious" balance with athletes. I think this is key to developing trust. I'm about getting the basics right. I think there's a way I deal with people and a way that I deal with players. It's bringing nutrition back to something simple that shows reward, in most cases, increases in performance. If I were a Premier League football player, would I really want to sit there and talk about nutrition, food and changing things? That's the perception that I think many elite players have about nutritionists. I always have this in mind: if an athlete enjoys how someone works with them, they'll buy into their practice.

I work with athletes in a personal, friendly way. I like to laugh with them. I want to have banter with them and make them relaxed. The first five minutes of a meeting is talking about something completely random, like what are they watching on Netflix? How's their house move going? What did they do on their day off? When you build a relationship with that player, they want to open up to you.

You'll know James, wherever you go, that you get a couple of players who are a bit standoffish; they think, what's this guy all about? I have a personality type that works in an environment other people, higher up, want to create. They want to create a relaxed atmosphere with good people. I like to think I try to be a good person, and that builds trust.

That brings me back to the first ever role I got at Hull City FC; even though the other interviewees knew a lot more than me and had more experience than me, I was brought in because they felt that my personality fit that environment. It's not just about "being nice"; the players know that when I'm serious, I'm serious. It's about being personable and understanding people, but it's also about not being scared to have difficult conversations when you must. That's important.

I try to get inspiration from sport psychologist Michael Caulfield, whom I initially worked with at Hull City FC and, more recently, at Brentford

Football Club. He is the most personable person I've ever met. He is unbelievable at what he does because you want to open up to him. Mike doesn't do fancy presentations, questionnaires with the players or anything like that, but after one conversation, you want to tell him your life story! That's what I want players to do, which is why I've succeeded.

I've worked hard academically, got my qualifications, and have a good base of scientific knowledge, but I wouldn't say I know anything more than any other practitioner. It's the way I try to put that across to clients. I think it's harder to get that than you think. I believe many nutritionists feel they've got to go in somewhere and demonstrate their knowledge and almost try to be too strict. We're not in these roles to go in there and change the world in a month. We're here to develop people slowly. Rome wasn't built in a day, and neither are athletes.

**What's been the biggest challenge of your career to date?**

**Ted:** Despite my strengths as a practitioner, I've had many challenges when working with certain people, whether athletes themselves or other backroom staff members. For example, there are certain places I've previously been where specific coaches or other members of the performance department want to know everything about players. They want to know exactly what their body composition data is, and they want to know the conversations we've been having. I used to share a lot of that on demand about a player, and I think I lost trust with some athletes because I was sharing too much about them with people they didn't want me to share that with.

At the time, I was thinking of a multidisciplinary approach with different practitioners, and I think that's what we're all taught, but I do think you've got to know what the player is like as a person and always ask, can I share this? Nutrition can be deeply personal to certain people, and we must respect that.

When a player comes to you and says, "I want to build some muscle", I'll share this with those that need to know, like the strength & conditioning coach (S&C) coach, head of performance etc. They're vital stakeholders, but I feel it's essential to keep some data between the nutritionist and the athlete, and this is down to the athlete's discretion. Sometimes in the past, I've had challenges where senior staff asked me personal things about an athlete. Some environments even have body composition leaderboards on the wall. Perhaps the player didn't want me to share that because they didn't want that to be used as a selection tool. It's striking that balance between what to share and what to keep to yourself, provided the player is developing their habits and behaviours.

There's been a few situations there, and probably, because of that, I found it a challenge with certain athletes that don't buy into your approach. I've seen athletes that don't want to be involved with the nutritionist. These athletes often don't get injured, stay the same weight, body comps are great, etc., but don't have that high-performance lifestyle. I worry about how that may influence other players. Will others see athletes' success and think they don't need nutrition support? Maybe they focus on nutrition but don't like to say it! I've dealt with a few athletes like that, and they influence younger players into that mindset of "Oh, I don't need to try so hard". That's a challenge, and maybe it comes back to trust. It can be harder to gain confidence from some players than others, and nobody is the same! There always comes a time for you to help that athlete. Maybe they pick up a strain, or their fitness scores drop. That's when, as a practitioner, you've got to demonstrate what you can do to help them.

## What characteristics do you think people need to work in performance nutrition as an industry?

**Ted:** Let's break down the characteristics. The number one characteristic that new or aspiring practitioners need to nail is that knowledge and developing that scientifically sound background, which you need to get at university. So, we've already discussed having that personality or way of adapting to a specific environment. This aspect comes with time and experience in different settings and requires making (and learning from) mistakes. I firmly believe that to provide nutrition advice (to athletes), you should attend a university and do courses endorsed by the British Dietetic Association (BDA) or Sport and Exercise Nutrition Register (SENR).

If you want to work in an elite sport, do not waste time with these courses that last six months and give you an accreditation; they miss out on many of the scientific fundamentals of physiology and anatomy. When I was at university, I thought, "I'm not going to use this..." but you do! It is the base of everything, the bottom of understanding. Ensure you are getting what is needed on the SENR graduate register.

Then there is the ability to coach people. That's something that I'm working on now, is how I coach people and be more of a leader. There are various ways to look at that and various ways to do that. I think we naturally have some leadership skills at varying levels. I don't think I've ever been anywhere where I've had a nutritionist above me for me to get advice from. Maybe that's because we got into sports nutrition early in our careers, but we need leadership and people to learn from. For example, many students will be jumping into a League One, League Two football team and need a leader above them. They might have a head of performance, but they're left to do their thing regarding nutrition support.

How do we make people do what we want them to do? There's human behaviour and how, as nutritionists, we can influence it. People should read up on that, understand their style and learn how to work with people. This ability comes from a mixture of your personality, demonstrating your knowledge, understanding situations and the athlete.

Nutritionists need to be able to persuade people to try things out and be able to show them progression. Finally, we've got to have excellent computer skills. For example, creating a pivot chart quickly to show a player or coach how muscle mass increases. Being able to "whip up" some eye-catching infographics or player feedback reports is essential. Some nutrition students I've worked with haven't had that ability on a laptop, and I've always told them to put themselves in an athlete's shoes. You want that feedback report to be clear, concise and presented well. The impact of technology will increase even more, and think about where we will be in five years, and we need to use it to our advantage.

**What are the most significant recommendations for your younger self or students entering nutrition now?**

**Ted:** For students entering nutrition now, I recommend exploring other aspects of sports science to help their nutrition work. I did the Catapult (Global Positioning System) level 1 course and my level 3 Football Association Physical Performance Award at St George's Park in the United Kingdom. These are two of the best practices I've ever done, and I think learning all of them has helped me better understand physical demands, coaching and other performance practitioners I work with.

On reflection, I would put more time into the coaching side of things at the start. Striking that balance, between 80% on scientific papers, 20% on behaviour change models, and some reading on leadership and coaching. I read my first leadership book during the lockdown. I wish I'd explored that earlier because it helps me put my ideas and knowledge out there and helps me deal with people depending on their learning styles.

We deal with so many people, and sometimes we don't have much time with them all. If we have 10 to 15 minutes with that person, how do we get what we want across in an easily manageable way that they understand? I want them to leave me thinking they've better understood than 15 minutes ago. I would have focused more on that when starting.

Right now, a practitioner only sometimes focuses on elite sports. Often, people message you and say they want elite experience, to work with the elite athlete in the Premier League, or to work with Premiership Rugby players. As someone who actively employs practitioners, I wouldn't mind if a junior practitioner didn't have experience at the highest level of elite sport.

I'd look to see if they have experience working with semi-pro teams and experience delivering an education programme. Do I care if it's working with a Premiership team or a division six football team... no. You've still got experience in an athletic setting.

Delivering education to a division six semi-professional team is more challenging because you'll get many more questions. You will be challenged to make it easy to understand because they might not have had any education before.

Don't focus your time chasing the Premier League football teams for the experience; can you go to your local swimming club or semi-professional football team and offer to help with a couple of people? You're more likely to learn a lot more and gain more experience. From my perspective, it's gaining time in an environment, delivering, and developing relationships. Shadowing is essential, and you can learn a lot in elite environments, but in terms of gaining experience, focus on something other than the elite.

Finally, another advice is to look at all aspects of sports science. One of the best things I've had is understanding GPS data. I was lucky to work with sports scientist Steve Barrett at Hull City when I started. He taught me a lot about GPS. I still put time into it today, most recently learning from Matt King at Brentford Football Club. It helps me determine things like calorie expenditure and helps individualise some of the practices I put in place. Is their load high? Have they done a lot of high-speed running, accelerations, and decelerations? This helps me with periodic nutrition for the athletes and determining various recovery methods throughout their training cycle. From my perspective, data is essential.

When you land that role, always work closely with the other performance practitioners in your team/organisation – they can significantly help you. I've spoken to some practitioners who thought they were alone in their team – just focusing on their cog in the big machine. For example, I catch up with our sports psychologist about how our players feel. Would they be up for a chat today? What's going on that may influence their nutrition behaviours? Sleep and nutrition are heavily linked. I've recently started working with a sleep specialist called Anna West. Learning from Anna has added a new tool to my toolbox and made me a better practitioner. So yeah, try to understand all aspects of sports science and don't just focus on the nutrition side. Even if it's just putting two hours aside a week to read something on sleep and performance, something you might not be getting taught in the course, it will help you in the long term.

Developing this whole rounded approach to sports science and performance will help you in interviews as well, because the person interviewing you may be the head of the department. If you can demonstrate that knowledge, that will put you a foot above the rest.

**This combines into the next question regarding the content you're not generally taught on a sports science course.**

**Ted:** One of my favourite modules at university was science and coaching pedagogy, which is the art and science of how to coach. That interested me. It was convenient, and you'd learn how to coach different people – like speaking to athletes, coaching methods, and other personality traits. I would implement this into any practical sports science or sport and exercise nutrition-related course. There are also many practical courses that you could jump on that aren't that expensive, such as Catapult level 1.

Nowadays, you must go out and seek that additional CPD. I was interested in tennis coaching back in the day, and I did my level 2 coaching badge. I learned how to coach people's skills the first time they picked up the racquet. I also learned leadership skills that I don't think my course offered. So, it doesn't always have to be a sit-at-home laptop course. If you're interested in something, you might also get some work out of it. I know of a tennis coach who started coaching, doing a sports science degree alongside his coaching. He got a job with the Lawn Tennis Association as a sports scientist – he combined his coaching and sports experience with his degree. You ask any practitioner how they gained their role, and I guarantee they have well-rounded sports science experience and a network. When you're at university, you've got to get networking with people. Many students come out of university with a master's and haven't spoken to anyone in the industry! I would certainly focus on networking.

**Where do you think the future of nutrition will be in five years?**

**Ted:** Individualisation still has a way to go. It can be tough to individualise nutrition depending on your time working with that group. Working one to one with an athlete is critical, but as technology improves, we will see even further individualisation. At the minute, we look at physical performance, tactical and even rehabilitation markers daily – but how are we focusing on individualisation with nutrition? Hopefully, we will see more practitioners (and research) focusing on sleep, gut health, and optimising health and performance.

We see athletes constantly on their phones and using technology – we must embrace it! I recently had a meeting with a company that analyses stool samples; the data we could get from it is eye-opening. It would allow us to learn more about individualised fuelling and recovery practices. I can see our field going down that route, but there will also be technological advances to help us with our daily role. For example, companies like Hexis are helping our athletes with education around periodisation – showing it in real time. Even companies like ZoneIn with the platforms help us write plans and get a better snapshot of food diaries to help us make quick recommendations.

I've always been a little bit traditional when communicating with athletes, just using WhatsApp, PDFs, voice notes, etc. But no matter what platform comes out, you'll always get the most from a conversation with your athlete, and we mustn't let technological advances take that away.

From a research perspective, it's great to see the quality and quantity of research increase since I was at university. I still think there are some ways we can go, certainly from different ways that we can look at that are less invasive, more field studies on things like calorie expenditures, physiological markers and easier ways to use technology. Even looking at the gut/brain axis and how different strains of probiotics could enhance recovery and aid sleep. I find that interesting.

So yeah, that's probably where we'll be in the next five years.

**Is there a book you've recently read which has improved your practice?**

**Ted:** The one that jumped out to me that I enjoyed was *Peak: The New Science of Athletic Performance* by Dr Marc Bubbs.

I read that last year after a recommendation. They dive into things that I could be more knowledgeable about. Things like sleep, digestion, and microbiome, and I like looking at how other people create nutrition strategies for specific goals like muscle build and fat loss. You've got to have an open mind when reading other practitioners' ideas and theories, and don't get me wrong; I don't implement every idea into my practice.

I read *Coaching for Performance* by John Whitmore in lockdown. I was looking at coaching books that develop potential leadership, which kept popping up, so I decided to get it. They introduce the "Grow Model" to structure how you coach people. You assess your client's **goals**, the **reality** of them completing the tasks, the **options** they have, and **the will** they have to do it. That stuck with me, and I try to link back to it when I work with athletes, but I always take those models with a pinch of salt!

Indeed, when I work with a new athlete or even an athlete with a new goal, I think: Okay, how could this athlete grow? Is what I'm asking them to do realistic? What sort of options do they have available to them? Do they have the kind of environmental factors around them? Can they cook? Do they have a support network at home? Do they have the will to do it, or are they being told? What motivates them?

At the moment, I'm really into podcasts, but I'm picky at what I listen to. Sometimes I find podcasts full of misinformation about nutrition, like social media. At Brentford Football Club, our director of elite performance is called Ben Ryan, and I knew him from his podcast "The Ben Ryan Podcast". He interviews high-end, successful people in the performance world and discusses culture, people like Stuart Lancaster and Craig White – exciting people with many experiences. I've been focusing a lot on that. You may as well get some learning in when you drive as much as I do!

**Are there any fundamental principles you try to follow daily to keep Ted Munson operating?**

**Ted:** Indeed. With me, I'm a contractor, and I have my own company. So I need to work as hard as I can day in, day out. I ensure everything is backed by science, even though sometimes I need to check myself a little! This is a key fundamental. However, we've also got to be innovative. We sometimes forget about that. In some instances, we need to think, okay, will it hurt to try this out? Could it have a benefit, and is anyone else doing it? It's okay to be the first to make some approach or try something different. Perhaps trying a new supplement with an athlete, as long as it's safe and tested and doesn't decrease performance – will it hurt? Are there potential performance gains? We need to strike that balance between being 100% science backed and being innovative. Not everybody is the same, so that's key.

I try to understand the person I'm working with and my environment because it can change daily. When we see people in the morning, as performance nutritionists, we first say, "How are you?" What's the response that you get? Is it "Okay"? What if they didn't seem okay? Or perhaps they say they had a hard time after a loss on the weekend? This should gauge how we work with that individual today. We've got to understand the person first and how they change all the time, just like we do as people. And that's how we go about working with them.

**In your opinion, and with your thoughts and experiences, what makes a successful performance nutritionist?**

**Ted:** I want to avoid repeating myself but get that sound scientific understanding that underpins everything we do. Question it, revisit it and develop it. If you need more clarification, reaching out to people is easy. Sometimes I was uncertain about a particular subject or theory, and I've done my best to reach out to an expert in that field to help me. For example, I was lucky to cross paths with David Dunne, whose PhD was in behavioural design thinking and technological innovation. I see him as an expert in his field. There have been multiple times I've asked him for advice on dealing with certain athletes, some of whom we'd both worked with in previous roles. It's straightforward to reach out to different people, so make sure you do that. Don't be scared because even the best ask for advice, you know? So, make sure that you dial in that science and continue developing that knowledge.

You've also got to invest time in coaching people and being an all-around good person that athletes want to open up to. Also, understand that only some people always want to talk about nutrition. So how can you make food exciting and fun? How can you show progression for people? That's important. For example, rather than just showing an athlete their sum of eight skinfold measurements, it's... How are you progressing? Always bring it down to the athletes' terms – how will it help them be better? Because that is why 99.9% of athletes see us; they want to be better, and that's how you'll be successful.

**Thank you, Ted.**

## JAMES'S THOUGHTS

When reading Ted's chapter, an area which stood out for me is his work with Science in Sport. SiS is a global sport nutrition supplement company and one which allowed Ted to network widely in sport. The power of your network is very important for your career and I would advise you to build your own network as widely as you can.

Another lesson from Ted is not taking too much on when running your own business! A lesson I am still learning myself. As Ted mentions, it can be tempting to apply for and say yes to as many contracts as possible, but you quickly realise that either you cannot manage the contracts, or your quality of work drops.

I love the idea Ted talks about in regard to learning off others: ensuring you have mentors in your career and also creating WhatsApp groups to share ideas. This is one of the main reasons I set up The Performance Nutrition Network.

Finally Ted makes a really good point about fundamental academics. If you want to be a credible, knowledgeable practitioner, you need to study a well-recognised undergraduate and master's course. Courses at this level will give you the core underpinning knowledge required to land most jobs in sports nutrition.

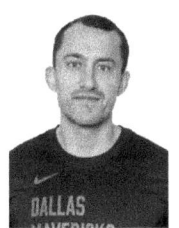

# CHAPTER 4:
# CHARLES ASHFORD

Charles is the performance nutritionist to National Basketball Association team Dallas Mavericks and was previously the director of sport nutrition at the University of North Texas.

Although it feels like I know Charles so well, incredibly we have never met in person! I knew of Charles and the great work he was doing over in America as a practitioner.

During COVID, Charles successfully set up and delivered a global online performance nutrition conference. I was so impressed with the first one that I offered to get involved and help with the second and subsequently trilogy conferences. Between the second and third conferences we raised over £12,000, donating it all to COVID charities, a charity close to the unfortunate 2020 Beirut explosion, and funding two students to study their master's in sports nutrition at university.

Since then Charles and I have stayed in touch and often send voice notes to update each other on how we are getting on in sport and business. It was an absolute privilege to interview Charles for this book and I know many will take inspiration from the journey he has gone on from the UK to USA.

You can follow Charles on:
Twitter @cashford_

**Who are you for those who need to be made aware of who you are? What is your background?**

**Charles:** I am Charles Ashford. I've been living in the US now for almost nine years. I was born and raised in High Wycombe in the UK. I went through the typical UK pathway to sports nutrition. I started with an undergrad degree in sports and exercise sciences. Then immediately after my degree I moved to the US. I currently serve as the performance nutritionist for the Dallas Mavericks in the NBA, residing in Dallas, Texas.

Having spent much time in the US and growing up with my dad, my dad did much business out here, so I always wanted to live and work in the US one day. As we know, it is very competitive and few and far between and I wanted to get hands-on experience. I was fortunate enough to get an internship with Texas Tech University, working with their American football team. It was unpaid, but my dad told me I had a year to see if I could make something work, and he helped me a little. They created a full-time position for me at the end of my first year there, so I started getting some income there. I spent the best part of three years at Texas Tech, which was a valuable experience. I was then super fortunate to have the opportunity to move to the University of North Texas, where I served as their director of sports nutrition; I moved there in 2017 and spent five years building a sports nutrition programme, which was a huge learning experience. I got the role at 23, which I wasn't ready for. I had the opportunity to build the staff, build a programme, and see all the inner workings of a collegiate athletics programme here in the US, which is a different level compared to what we're used to in the UK university scene. From there, I was approached by the Dallas Mavericks out of nowhere with an opportunity to come on board as their first full-time performance nutritionist and build a nutrition programme within the organisation, and that's where I am currently.

**How and when did you first get involved in nutrition? Could you give some insight there on your academics as well?**

**Charles:** Yeah, during my undergrad degree, I was still playing sports and beginning to train myself and take more of an interest in what I was doing from a nutrition standpoint. Around the same time, I was going through my first year of university, and some of these exercise physiology classes and different courses piqued my interest. There is much information online, typical bro science, bodybuilding magazines and exposure to better communication. I even looked towards famous guys within that physique industry, like Alan Aragon and Eric Helms, that share a sound evidence base and sources of information. I found it fascinating.

It wasn't until that first year when I met with my advisor, Dr Carl Hulston, who was at Brunel University at the time, that I realised that sports nutrition was an avenue or career. I walked into his office with many different supplements, and he spoke about some of the studies and their work.

From that moment on, this is what I wanted to do. I was getting exposed to the academic level and building my base level of knowledge but then spending a lot of my time looking at what I believe are good sources of information and building my knowledge base, and then discussing this with friends. I mean, I just became obsessed, honestly. From then on, I started to look at how I could better tailor my degree to fit the needs of what I was looking to do and align that with postgraduate study. I had several offers from UK master's programmes, and I decided that Leeds Beckett University would be my next step. About a week before the start of the degree programme, I got the green light to go to Texas, so I pulled the plug on the master's and moved to the US. There was probably a two or three-week period during my undergrad where this idea of going in and wanting to be a sports coach was utterly turned on its head, and now sports nutrition was everything; that's what I wanted to do from a career standpoint.

**So, the turning point was your father getting the job in America, which meant you moved over there? Is that right?**

**Charles:** No, this goes back to being as young as at primary school when my dad was making trips to the US for business, taking me out of school, and spending time over here. During the school year, during the summer holidays, I often returned to the US. During the end of my undergrad degree, the girl I was dating at the time did a year abroad in San Diego. I'd made a couple of trips to the US, and it was almost like, wow, I love being out here. Can I get myself back out here? As I finished my undergrad degree, I started exploring opportunities. I'm emailing and applying for jobs where I need more experience and the qualifications to get involved. Fortunately, I stumbled across an internship opportunity which was meant for university students at that time. But the person who had put the posting out had reached out to me and tried to gain an understanding of what I was trying to do. I explained that I was fresh from undergrad and wanted to pursue sports nutrition as a career pathway. This was before the days of Zoom.

We had several Skype calls and got to know each other briefly. At the end of that summer, before the master's programme was due to begin, they told me if you want to do this, you can come over. We can sponsor a visa for a year and see where that takes us. I dropped everything to go and do that. In hindsight, I look back on it, it's kind of crazy to just up and leave at the age of 21 to move halfway across the world with no guarantee of anything. The agreement was a year. We speak today almost nine years on from that point. It's neat to see the development and still be here.

**Yeah, it's a crazy background. You said that at 23/24, you were asked to build that strategy within your first role at the college. We'll come on to that a little bit more later. But you know, such a young practitioner there, to be asked to do that is incredible. Before we come into that, who were or are some of the most significant mentors in your life? Why have they been essential for you too?**

**Charles:** Like most, you always have a family member that you lean towards. For me it's my dad; his work ethic is unbelievable. Even at his current age, he has always shown a fantastic work ethic in his day to day and always provided for us, and I am fortunate to have inherited a fraction of that. Even the time we spent in the US growing up laid the foundations for me. Even then, in those first couple of years when I was alone and young and had doubts about being here, he reassured me that this was where I needed to be. If I got myself in trouble financially, you know, not making a whole lot at the time, he would bail me out for a bit and tell me to stick with it, and now it's cool, and it's come full circle, and he's visiting maybe two or three times a year since COVID has passed. He takes much pride in seeing what I'm doing and being involved in that, and I owe a lot to him. I would probably have packed it in a few years ago without him.

I would also say my boss at Texas Tech University, Dayna McCutchin. I was sending these emails without much luck and much response, and she got back to me and took an interest in what I was trying to do. It gave me the green light and support to come out here, and a mum away from home; she always took care of me, even at a period when I wasn't making any money, always made sure I had food, had a ride wherever I need to go when I didn't have a car, would involve me in her family holidays, when I had no family over here. I will always appreciate that, not only from the human side but also from what she showed me. She was building a programme herself, and seeing the rate at which it developed and the backing she got as we grew our sports nutrition programme was a fantastic experience and helped prepare me for taking a position down the line, and I would be responsible for that.

When my time came, she was disappointed to let me go, but she co-signed on my competency as a practitioner and gave the green light to the new employer that I could do the job. I was a lot younger than most in getting that opportunity, but she believed in me and not only gave me that opportunity but allowed me to move on from there. So, I owe her a lot. From there, I would say, especially in this career transition phase, getting to work with some individuals: our current performance director, Jeremy Holsopple. Then even a fellow Brit, Jeremy Bettle, who spent several years in the US in elite sport, just having inside knowledge of people with a wealth of experience and professional sport, making you aware of your blind spots and giving you actionable feedback is incredibly powerful. Sometimes in this field, we focus so much on the knowledge aspect; but just how you interact with people, how you communicate with athletes, and having their insights has helped me view how I operate differently in this space. Those guys have been hugely valuable to my development this past year.

Nice. That's excellent insight there. If I were to ask you, what's been a standout moment for your career today? Is there anything that jumps out? Or are there a few things?

**Charles:** Yeah, personally and professionally, it's getting that role at North Texas. My time to leave Texas Tech had approached, and almost a perfect opportunity arose for me at the right time. Although I was out of my depth, we had much success in our football programme those first few years. This was a brand-new programme being delivered to these athletes from a team which had yet to have much success a few years prior, but there was almost this feeling of all hands on deck from support staff to the administration. We were winning games.

We had a great group of athletes whose interest in nutrition was high as this was brand new. It helped me a lot, especially as I was learning the ropes of the position, to have a group that was engaged and interested in what we were trying to do. So not only did we make a lot of successes and strides day to day, but we were also seeing a lot of positive results on the field, which helped the momentum of the programme, and we were able to get more investment quickly. The administration realised that this programme was going somewhere and was putting the resources forward to support the athletes. The athletes appreciated that especially being a new programme they hadn't had before. Maybe I didn't enjoy it as much then, but now I look back on that and take much pride in having the opportunity to build that programme and having an engaged group. It was a great experience.

**Would you have received the funding and the support if the on-field performances weren't there?**

**Charles:** If I am being honest, probably not, not at the rate we did. We had the perfect storm across teams and sports; nutrition was a brand-new piece of the puzzle. We were having the on-field results in football; being in Texas, college football holds much weight. We got lots of backing quickly; fortunately, all sports benefited from that. However, I would like to remind people that nutrition plays a small part in those moments. But then it also taught me, as a practitioner, mainly operating in that environment, when I could push a little bit and go to the administration and ask for the things I thought necessary to develop and grow as a programme. Whereas, as I went through my career, I was having to be more strategic when I did that, learning to know when you can strike a little, when you can get away with asking for things and seeing where you may have to be a little more reserved. I was leaning on the key stakeholders and understanding the broader ecosystem within an organisation beyond just nutrition. So, I don't think we got the backing that we did so quickly. But that made the transition easier for me. Again, the athletes saw some of those immediate benefits and impacts we could make, which coincided with my employment and being there. That helped me get that buy-in quickly.

**Yeah, and anyone who's worked in a team sport knows that when the wins are there, you've got to take them, grab them, and make sure you enjoy them. What is it that you've got that other nutritionists or dietitians in the States may not have, or what is something that you've been able to bring to the party? What do you think has been the most influential factor as to why you've been successful today?**

**Charles:** Yes, that's a tough one, an ability to be proactive, take a bit of a risk, and maybe do some things others are unwilling to do. I was moving to a foreign country at a young age and putting myself out there. As I said, looking back at it at the time it seemed risky. But I needed to take that risk to have the opportunities I've had in my career. I know this is only possible for some. The circumstances differ for each practitioner, but I created an opportunity that didn't exist. I took something that wasn't there, which evolved into a full-time role. Even my current position only existed after I came on board. Taking a chance and then being authentic. I genuinely think back to those undergrad days being passionate about the field. I'm passionate about improving my knowledge and am generally interested in performance nutrition. I don't think you can fake that.

Being authentic and genuine is such a massive part of daily practice. When I meet or interact with people in the field, those with a true passion for nutrition rise to the top and achieve what they want in the space and the area. Having had the opportunity to hire and interview several individuals over the years, that shines through quickly. It shines through to athletes too. We always speak about someone being the most knowledgeable person in the world. Still, if they are not good human beings, their chances of being practical and communicating are almost zero. So that shines through.

Lastly is networking advice. It doesn't have to be with other nutritionists, dietitians, or people in performance roles. I know this gets spoken about a lot, but being genuine builds genuine connections with others and does not underestimate any interaction you have.

As the years have passed, I realise how small the infrastructure is in sports. Who knows who has been where and whose paths have crossed. A few weeks ago, someone told me it's not who you know but who knows you, which remarkably stuck with me.

The individual who had passed on my name for this position was someone I'd never met before, but they were aware of my work from someone else. So again, always appreciate the power of your network and your interactions. Everything from how you present yourself on social media and how you present yourself in day-to-day interaction, regardless of if that's with a general manager or another member of your support staff or someone you may meet informally, on a road game or something and have a brief interaction with, you never know where people end up. So just be mindful of that. I think just having a genuine connection in your networking, not just hitting people up asking for jobs or opportunities when those opportunities arise, just being yourself, and being approachable, goes a long way.

**Yeah, mate, that's awesome. I finished Louise Burke's interview the other day and asked her, "What's one of your most significant recommendations to those entering the industry now?" She said, being creative. There weren't jobs for her when she started; she made her own roles. There are opportunities that people can have an adventure on. It's just continually looking for little opportunities, backing yourself to do it, and then having patience.**

**That sounds like your career.**

**Charles:** Even getting the job at North Texas, the offensive coordinator for the football team was a Hall of Fame player for Texas Tech, and he called our equipment manager about me. It was just a character recommendation, nothing concerning how I work or operate. That is something to remember when you go through your interactions. You never know who your biggest advocate on the other end could be or maybe be the roadblock between you and that kind of final hurdle.

**What's been the biggest challenge of your career to date?**

**Charles:** We can return to that standout moment and remind ourselves that nutrition doesn't necessarily dictate wins and losses. Take a step back and understand that nutrition plays a small role in building success, but many other factors go into that. I found it challenging during some points in my career when I was putting in a lot of time, hours, and effort, which may not match the results – so taking that a little bit personally. What else can I do, or what else could I do better?

Try not to take those tough times personally. Also, finding ways to detach from work, especially now that the hours are extended in a professional sports environment, and there are few days off. Many times, you wait to know your day-to-day schedule. Work does come first often, and just finding ways to disengage when possible outside of work. It's probably something which has helped me and my career to date or being so involved and interested in what I do – but having the ability to take a step back sometimes, that I don't solely identify as a performance nutritionist. I am a husband and have other hobbies and interests outside of work. I am reminding myself that the world still spins. So, that has been challenging for me throughout my career and something I'm still working through myself.

Then lastly would be the wins and losses. It's understanding that only some athletes will be super engaged or interested in nutrition from the off. For some guys, their external or internal motivation is different, especially across a team with different ages, backgrounds, and upbringings; only some athletes are the same. Sometimes things take time. Although you have all this excellent knowledge you want to impart to athletes, you believe you can help them.

One, not being so hard on myself in that sense, but two, reminding myself I must try to engage and interest them. Whereas I felt early in my career, if the athlete doesn't care, that's on them; that should be within their interests. Therefore, I'll let them do their own thing.

Well, now I have more of a mindset where if I have an athlete where the interest levels are not there, I am looking for different ways to engage them, and almost making it a challenge to myself or finding a way for me to measure my skill set as a practitioner to try and engage that athlete. Early in my career, I look back, and some athletes may have felt like I didn't give them a chance in that sense.

A recent example was when I was invited back to my previous role to speak to some undergraduate student-athletes at a career night and some of the athletes from a team I'd worked with. We had a cordial interaction, but there wasn't a significant interaction, and they were probably athletes I put off into that bucket that they didn't care and weren't interested. So I gave them less time or not as much attention as I would give to the interested guys.

In hindsight, if I'd done more of that, I could have captured them, built a better relationship with them, and got them to follow through on the stuff I wanted them to do instead of writing them off so early. Now I see it as a challenge, and athletes respect that if you do it in a way that their best interests are there. You're genuine that you're trying to help them. Eventually, those barriers will come down, and you can reach them. Some athletes take longer than others. So that was a humbling reminder, even seeing some of these athletes and individuals down the line, thinking back to that.

**It's the problematic athletes that I sometimes find, when you get them to buy into it eventually, and they get it, they're the enjoyable case studies that you learn so much about because you know what it was that you've worked on now with them that's allowed them to then buy into it.**

**What characteristics do you think people need to work in our field? You know what the nutrition field is like in the UK, but you've also got this wealth of knowledge and experience of what it's like stateside.**

**Charles:** Something I've spoken about already. I think it's just being genuine and being approachable. Nutrition is still a pretty niche area regarding performance support. In the US, their strength conditioning coach gets much hands-on time with athletes, whereas in nutrition, you don't have accurate, hands-on scheduled times; being approachable and enjoyable to be around for athletes is critical.

Something that's been a challenge to me is having self-confidence in these environments to approach athletes in different environments. You could be the most intelligent person in the world, but if you're at the laptop all day, making meal plans, and infographics, many times athletes will miss out and not seek you out. You must find opportunities to get these interactions in because you must schedule time in the training room. You don't have scheduled time in the weight room.

A professional athlete only has a little time throughout the day. So, it would be best if you found those opportunities. But as my career's gone on, a lot of this comes back to the ability to build genuine relationships with athletes. Being open and approachable is something that now, if you'd asked me this a few years ago, probably wouldn't have been near my first response.

So being approachable is a big one. Being in an elite environment with many moving parts, being organised and having an eye for detail is critical. It can only take one small mistake or oversight to lose the trust of athletes or even stakeholders in your group. It's often the work that some practitioners may take for granted, some of the logistic work. The team is currently on a week-long road trip; many meals are scheduled there, and many moving parts.

Being proactive about that and having an eye for detail is essential. A good example would be some of the roles in the UK, many practitioners aren't full time with their teams, but you can build much trust by being organised, having an eye for detail, and not giving stakeholders or your supervisor an excuse to have to call you out on things.

Being coachable is essential. That's a straightforward way to help build trust in those environments. Also, being able to take feedback, seek feedback, and get other people's perceptions of your work. The way you operate is so valuable. I should have done more early in my career. Even though I'm closing in on a decade of applied work, this year has probably been the year I've developed the most as a practitioner. That's little to do with the knowledge I'm gaining or the reading I'm doing. It's about how I operate with athletes and how to communicate. All these things are so important in being effective in your role.

I had a few shortcomings in roles which I thought would come together for me in the last couple of years. Being coachable, being able to take feedback and looking at ways to develop those soft skills can set a young practitioner apart. Lastly, persistence. I was being persistent with athletes, who were only partially there regarding their interest or readiness to change, but also in trying to acquire and obtain roles.

I was persistent, and I stayed the course. I was ready to make the jump to work in elite sports. When that opportunity arose, I took some feedback I got on those interviews and tried to apply it to the day to day. I was persistent in my work and believed my opportunity would come if I continued doing things correctly daily.

In a field where it is very competitive, these roles only pop up now and then. If you're persistent and want it, that will shine through in the interview process. This attitude will carry you into your day-to-day work too.

Even now, I have days where I question what I'm doing here; I might need help to get buy-in or be compliant with certain things, and then the next day looks completely different. So, it's understanding that if you bring that positive attitude and work ethic daily, things will work out okay.

**I'm diverging a little bit. But you mentioned the team travelling so much now. Are you the person that writes the menus, or have you got the chef that does that, and then you work with the chef to create the meal plans?**

**Charles:** A combination of both; the chef does much of our airline catering. When we fly out of Dallas, our kitchen serves the aircraft. We own our plane, we have the same flight attendant crew, and the chef will coordinate the menu, prepare the food, and deliver it to the aircraft from our training facility. When the team is on the road, I work with a third party to coordinate the food for the plane. Between the lead flight attendant and myself, we will work with him. He will identify a restaurant, he may send us a sample menu, we'll make the changes that we believe necessary, different dietary restrictions on the plane, make sure that's handled, and they will deliver the food to the aircraft, my flight crew will take the delivery and provide the menus on the plane.

At the hotels, I'm responsible for the menus. So I am working with our travel coordinator. Whenever we're normally operating two to three weeks out from a stay, the hotel manager reaches out, I would typically ask for some kind of catering or banquet guide that the hotel offers. Fortunately, we stay at friendly hotels, and they often have pretty good culinary teams.

I will formulate the menus from there. So we provide breakfast, lunch and dinner every day on the road. On a game day, we provide breakfast, lunch, and pre and post-game meals; breakfast and the pre-game meal mostly stay the same. Trying to find a variety of lunches and dinners can be challenging sometimes. With a minimum of 41 road games over the season, there are many hotel stays. But having done enough now, it doesn't take too long, but again, going back to that logistic point and having an eye for detail, it's more of an understanding and something that must be done. Is it a favourite part of my job? No, but it helped gain some buy-in around what we do. Previously, it had always been left to another member of the support staff who maybe doesn't have experience or expertise in curating menus or understanding different fields, how to set up a buffet on the road, some of the different foods that go together and go well together. Now the guys are seeing different foods and different menus and get to experience other things.

In the grand scheme of things, trying to control their intake and get them to achieve the intakes we want without those meals would probably be challenging. It's a big logistical piece, but I have it under control now.

**So what would be your biggest recommendation to your younger self or students entering the industry now?**

**Charles:** Getting hands-on experience as early as possible is critical. This wasn't something I did during my undergrad degree. Fortunately, I got full-time work experience immediately out of my undergrad degree. So I was able to microwave that a little bit. Nothing could have substituted for that experience. I was getting interaction with athletes every day, and at the same time, I was able to enrol in the Institute of Performance Nutrition diploma (IOPN) when I first started at Texas Tech. So when I got home at night, I was self-studying. I was gaining this knowledge. Then the next day, I was back in the office and had the opportunity to apply it. I got to speak to my boss about it. We got to bounce ideas off each other, and it was a precious period for me. I wasn't just sitting at home, absorbing this content and material. I had a chance to apply and develop my understanding and some of the things we were doing daily.

You will get hit, and some people won't respond. You'll have to be proactive and look for opportunities and, much like you mentioned earlier, you can certainly make those opportunities. Having the persistence to create those is incredibly valuable. I'm still developing soft skills, I think. I've harped on about it a lot, too. When I first got a position in North Texas, I was pretty sure of my knowledge and that I was able to piece together a programme, but I did not understand the relationship with the business office, the administration, and all these key stakeholders, which was so crucial in me being successful. I didn't have an understanding or grasp of that. I probably hurt some of those relationships by coming in too aggressively.

As time went on, I understood how those relationships could help or hinder me. So one, working with others, and two, the athletes, as well, it's crucial in becoming an effective practitioner and probably something that I could have improved at earlier in my career. That is the focus of my development now, as I still look for ways to improve. When we look at young graduates entering the industry, there's a ton of excellent degree programmes, even undergrad degrees in sports nutrition, which were not a thing when you and I were in school. Graduate degrees are ideal. People are coming out with similar qualifications but looking for these ways to differentiate themselves. The ability to utilise stakeholders or relationships and get hands-on experience can set you apart early on.

What I like there that you've described is where you were doing the Texas Tech role. But then you'd go out of your way and out of your effort and motivation, you've then studied the IOPN in the evening when I imagine most people would be having beers and going to restaurants. Then you've almost described what I felt like on my PhD when I was in the club in the morning, and then in the afternoon, I was going to read journals or papers that were directly related to the conversations I was having the next day.

So what you've described there is so powerful because you get that experience, exposure and immersion of being involved with athletes while studying. I often say to the people on my mentorship programme that it doesn't have to be Chelsea Football Club straightaway; it doesn't have to be Warrington Wolves straightaway. It can be the local rugby club, and it could be the 16-year-old neighbour who's pretty nifty at golf but has got no idea about nutrition because the conversations you have with them at that level quite often are similar to conversations that you have with a team when you're in an organisation.

**Charles:** Just a few weeks ago, I was invited to a high school in the area to give a presentation to athletes' parents, and that was one of the hardest things I've done in the last few years. I work with some of the best athletes in the NBA daily, and I feel comfortable with that. But now, speaking to a guardian or provider for a child and trying to deliver some content is incredibly difficult. So never turn your nose up at experience or believe that it must be an elite or organised sport. You know, just having the ability to work with different individuals is compelling, especially when you're definitely marrying that education and applied piece.

**Are there any areas you did not learn on the course when you were studying that you feel have been essential to you now that you're working full time? Where are the gaps in some of the courses that students are covering?**

**Charles:** It's probably something that gets a little more focus in the dietetic degrees, this ability to counsel and look at the assessment and readiness to change, which I think are essential. I know this area has gotten much attention over the last couple of years with the work of some outstanding practitioners in the space of behaviour change. Again, I go back to some of those experiences earlier in my career where the athlete wasn't interested or seemed ready to get on board so that I would almost disregard them instead of looking for what I could do to capture them.

It's great that the BDA has a course right now where practitioners can sign up and participate in the workshop. Even right now, reading around this work, looking outside of a sports nutrition space and looking at the behaviour change and psychology literature is incredibly important. Those areas are essential. You probably see an underlying theme in this interview; I believe those things are vital to effectiveness.

My route in sports nutrition wasn't traditional; I didn't do the typical master's degree in sports nutrition immediately. Those early years of being embedded in the programme full time whilst studying every night, what I took out of those couple years was so valuable to me, and put me on the right path. It wasn't until later in my career that applied work was so powerful for me, which can often be sometimes lacking in the academic setting.

At the time, I was probably blind to it because I didn't pay as much attention to what I was doing at university until it was too late. So just having the opportunity to get applied hands-on experience is important for those who want to fast track their careers. Those opportunities exist a little bit more today as the field has grown. But anyway, the programmes can allow their students to get hands on with athletes. Fortunately, many of these schools which have excellent graduate programmes also have excellent sport scholar programmes. So if you are looking for those opportunities, I can't suggest it enough for young practitioners coming up.

**So where do you think the future of nutrition will be in five years?**

**Charles:** We're seeing AI coming down the pipeline, for better or worse; it's exciting. We were going to see this application in some way, shape or form in performance nutrition, and we already see that. There are ways that we can automate some different things to help decision-making and get us back to getting in front of the athletes and creating some of the opportunities we discussed previously. We may see a little bit more here in the US than in the UK: a performance nutritionist wearing multiple hats within an organisation, being a little bit more hands on with the strength and conditioning, sports science, and psychology piece. To be effective and an excellent performance nutritionist, you have to have a good understanding of those areas as it is.

There are a few practitioners over here in the US that have dual credentials (for example nutrition and strength and conditioning) and can operate in both spaces. I can say that spending a little bit of time in the weight room on the floor with athletes is a good time; maybe impart some nutrition knowledge and get good face time with athletes. So that'd be an excellent way to differentiate yourself and improve your value. As a practitioner, if you can wear multiple hats in an organisation and provide those services, chances are you will improve your worth. Lastly, we talk a lot about personalised nutrition approaches. I believe we'll take a step closer to having a better understanding of the tools that can help us prescribe some of that, whether that's biomarkers, the microbiome, DNA testing, or the use of constant glucose monitors; all these things still seem to be somewhat in their infancy, and I think we will take steps to be able to utilise those tools in applied practice better. We will have the opportunity to really create this personalised approach that a lot of us speak about and maybe have some better tools to deliver that in applied practice truly.

**So is there a book you've recently read which has improved your practice?**

**Charles:** Yes, I just finished *Nudge* by Richard Thaler and Cass Thunstein, going back to this behaviour change piece within shaping and influencing decision-making and how to steer individuals towards better choices. That's what we're trying to do daily as performance nutritionists. Relating to the previous question is *Range* by David Epstein, with this idea of having broader experiences and this interdisciplinary approach which is common to sports support staff. Nutrition is still a small area in that broader ecosystem. Understanding what you can bring to the table through S&C, sports science, and psychology – practitioners who grasp that tend to thrive, especially at the elite end of sports.

**What was the first book you mentioned?** *Nudge?* **What would be your one takeout from that?**

**Charles:** How can you subconsciously influence decision-making and choices? Even everything down to placing foods, supplements, or beverages in the facility. Looking at some of the studies and experiments they referenced in the book, with even just the labelling and the placements of different things, got me thinking about that practice facility. Something we've looked at trying to improve this year is compliance with the daily supplements; it's not so much that athletes don't want to take them, it's just they may get pulled in multiple directions, they may miss them, that one opportunity to see them each day, maybe they don't visit that area. So now we've set up our daily supplementation in the more high-traffic area where athletes must walk through multiple times a day. So there are almost numerous nudges without even realising that they take this up, purely just that switch alone without any additional education or follow-through on our end; we've seen an improvement in compliance. So even something which is out of sight, out of mind, all the time, just a little bit of fall behind, perhaps improving the placement of the salad or the fruits and vegetables in a dining hall. It's funny how quickly the consumption of those foods increases. I spoke about having an eye for detail and thinking about those things earlier. You'd be surprised how powerful it can be.

**Yeah, yeah. It's amazing. We've changed a few things around Bristol Bears. One example is whole fruit in a bowl being cut up into a fruit platter. It's prepped and ready, and all they need to do is grab it, whereas, for whatever reason, they don't want to eat the whole apple; they'd rather have slices. It's just a glaring example of where if you make it simple, stupid for people, they will buy into it.**

**Are there any fundamental principles that you try and follow every day?**

**Charles:** Yeah, this is a big one for me, especially something I've reminded myself of a lot this year, although my schedule is long. We work many consecutive days. When those athletes walk to the facility or spend time in the dining hall, you're one of the first people they see daily, and you can set the tone for that. Having a good attitude, putting aside what you have going on on the outside, showing up to work in a good mood, and carrying that good work ethic is just an old-fashioned cliched statement. I think it's something to not take for granted.

You never really know who's watching, so it's understanding that a good attitude and effort can go a long way. Something more for individuals further on in their career, a good reminder, even a habit to get into early in their careers, is taking care of yourself. We often spend so much time trying to improve the health and performance of others. It's easy to let your health and performance fall by the wayside slightly. So, taking time every day to do something for yourself and get physical activity in every day, something this year I've taken on is 10 to 15 minutes a day, actively trying to tune out a little bit, do a little bit of meditation, trying to protect my sleep where I can on non-game nights.

It's hard to show up daily with that good attitude and work ethic if you don't care for yourself. How are you meant to provide the best and highest level of service for athletes if you can't take care of yourself and are a walking example of that? So, remind yourself that your health and efforts can go a long way in supporting you daily. That's something I've had to remind myself of before. It's always interesting when you train more consistently and stay on top of your nutrition: your energy levels during the day and your energy and interactions improve significantly. All can play into being effective in your day-to-day role.

**Yes, it's so true. I was saying to my wife, I was looking at my next six weeks, and I think I've got something on every day. Because it's Red Roses, it's Bears, crunch time in the season. You know, I've got my business stuff going on and we've got Mila's birthday. I know when I'm getting overworked because two things happen: I get a stye, and then I'll get a cold**

sore. It's the first sign of my immunity beginning to take a dip. I know that. I need to, for the next six weeks, rip into it.

**Final question, in your eyes, what makes a successful performance nutritionist?**

**Charles:** Yeah, this is the million-dollar question. I pick an individual who can successfully influence and enable athletes to make good decisions around their health and performance. I know that's easier said than done. But a lot of what we've spoken about in the last couple of hours comes back to being a genuine, passionate, interested individual in this space. Being genuinely interested in the field and getting into it for the right reasons, and wanting to help individuals is the bottom line. You can accumulate and develop the knowledge as you go along. The practitioners I've got to work with, the practitioners I've hired, and the individuals I've seen operate in this field over the years, rarely do I see someone not have those kinds of critical skills. But if you don't have a genuine interest or passion for your work, I think you'll get found out quickly.

## JAMES'S THOUGHTS

If, like me, you have always wondered what professional sport would be like in America, for an English practitioner, now you have the answer. Since our first interactions during the COVID-19 conferences, Charles has become a close friend. I will often WhatsApp him asking his views on applied situations and see how it may differ or be the same in America.

Charles provides a great example of someone who is not afraid to take risks, put himself out there and do things that others might not want to do or feel comfortable doing.

A standout from this interview is when Charles received his character reference from someone whom he had never met before. However, importantly, this person was aware of Charles's work from someone else. This again shows the power of having a solid network but also being a good person in life. You never know who you meet and you never know who can speak positively or negatively about you! As you progress through your career, it is important to stay true to your values and be a respectful, honest and credible practitioner.

My final point from this chapter is the advice to get experience, volunteer and enjoy being proactive. There are so many athletes across the world who would love to have some education, advice or strategies to improve their performance; you just need to find them!

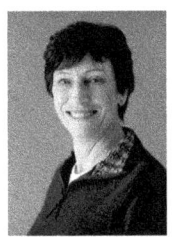

# CHAPTER 5:
# *RUTH WOOD-MARTIN*

Ruth spent 16 years with Irish Rugby as the head of nutrition. She has spearheaded a drive to build a department in Irish Rugby which has recruited six full-time and five part-time nutritionists. This is the biggest nutrition team in global rugby. Ruth is on the Healthspan Elite expert panel and also an assessor for the SENR.

I have never met Ruth personally but have always heard superb things about her work and passion for both rugby and nutrition. Having spent nine years working in professional rugby myself, it was a pleasure to interview Ruth for this book and listen to her path in sport.

You can follow Ruth on:
Twitter @WoodRwm

**So let's start with question one, in terms of your background. Where did it all start for Ruth Wood-Martin?**

**Ruth:** I was born in the west of Ireland on a farm, so food was always important, and we got reared on good, wholesome foods.

Science was my strong subject area so that, linked with the love of food and people, led me to study human nutrition and dietetics in Dublin back in the 1980s. My career has always been focused on nutrition, which is perhaps different from, I suppose, the mainstay of our profession in performance nutrition, where people are coming from a lot of different backgrounds. There's value in that on the one hand because it gives you possibly more diversity of science about exercise. However, studying nutrition and dietetics gives you the "whole-body" nutrition knowledge and application which is valuable in the world of nutrition education.

I worked in clinical and community dietetics up until 2006, doing some sports nutrition work along the way. But it was, as was the case back then, more dabbling than anything else. My first full-time role in sports nutrition was in 2006, with the IRFU (Irish Rugby Football Union). Before that, I worked with several athletes from various sports at the Sports Institute Northern Ireland. I worked with Irish Women's Hockey and that stemmed from the fact that my background in sports was hockey. I played international hockey, so I always had a link to sports and in particular a link to team sports.

I was one of the oldies who did the BDA accreditation in sports nutrition back in 1994. That's all that was available back then when you were working full time. There weren't the opportunities that there are now to study sports nutrition on a full-time or part-time basis as a postgraduate if you needed to keep working.

I grew my experience in sports nutrition after that. The "graduates" from this course were grand-parented over onto the Sport and Nutrition Register (SENR) when it became a live register in 2006. So that's who I am and what my background is.

**Yeah, that's awesome. It's amazing to think because there'll be people studying now that will not have a clue about 1994, BDA accreditation and nutrition and dietetics. So, it's really good to hear that because I want people to understand and highlight that there are these individuals that got our profession to where it is now. You know what I mean?**

**Ruth:** Yes, because it was from that that I think the first postgraduate certificate in Coventry was developed. It wasn't until probably the mid-2000s that a lot more postgraduate programmes at, for example, John Moores, Leeds Beckett, Westminster, University of Ulster in Ireland in Coleraine, evolved and developed. I remember talking at length with Graeme Close before he and James Morton developed the master's at John Moores (LJMU). An interesting part for them was, what can we offer at LJMU that has not been offered before? Even then, coming from a dietetic background, it was a valuable platform to understand the necessity to translate science into practice, because that's what dietitians do. That's their core business, to be able to interpret the science of nutrition to improve health and prevent and treat clinical diseases and conditions. It is that translation of science into practical eating and drinking if you like. So I said to him that that was one element that I felt in postgrad education that needed to be included. You're a graduate of there so you will be able to see the value in having that element within a master's programme.

**How and when did you first get involved in nutrition and potential research? I know you've spent years at Irish Rugby. Would you say that was your first real applied role or was there something before that?**

**Ruth:** Well, it's always been nutrition with me; I didn't come from a sports science background. Dietetics focuses on the role of nutrition in health, disease prevention, and condition management, and that is very valuable. But that's not enough to work in the field of sports nutrition and performance nutrition. But having that whole-body nutrition background is useful. I think practitioners now in the field of performance nutrition will just see how much health is playing a role in their work, gut health, for example, and conditions that the players will have, be it diabetes, be it bowel disorders. It's just becoming more and more common to encounter these conditions in athletes. So having that whole-body nutrition, education and knowledge has been fundamental for me. It's a great platform to move into performance nutrition; however, it's crucial to have further study to understand exercise physiology, and how nutrition impacts this is crucial to be competent to work in the field of sports nutrition.

So, at that time, back in 1994, that's what the BDA accreditation course did. Tutors included Clyde Williams and Ron Maughan, the godfathers of exercise metabolism. Being a dietitian is great, but you need more than that and I'm very clear on that to anybody in dietetics, who thinks they can leap into the world of sports nutrition. It's like any other speciality; it's like paediatric dietetics or cardiac dietetics. So it's a speciality. For me, what I needed to do was upskill and continue to upskill on exercise physiology and understand the impact that nutrition has on that.

Sharon Madigan and I provided nutrition services to the Sports Institute in Northern Ireland when it was set up in 2002. I worked with some athletes who would have been Olympic or Commonwealth athletes there, in hockey and athletics. I also worked at Irish Ladies' Golf. Then in 2006, the opportunity for a full-time role with the IRFU came up. To be fair to them, they were probably the first home nation to consider nutrition as a role. It's fair to say that the position was driven by the need to regulate supplement use, to be quite honest, as there was a lot of unregulated use going on with a lot of athletes at that time. This was 2006 and supplements were seen as being essential to succeed. I took up that post when I had 20 years of experience within clinical and community dietetics and from a sporting background and some sports work. It probably took that experience, both life and professional, to be equipped to take on that role.

I suppose in an elite performance environment and a male-majority sport, you do need to be able to hold your own professionally. You may come close to your professional boundaries; you feel out of your comfort zone. But I think what I would say to new practitioners is to trust your professional instinct, and it will not allow you to cross that line. But sometimes that's hard because there's pressure. So when I went into the IRFU in 2006, the position was in the medical department, which was great, because that was a professional setup which gave me support for an evidence-based approach.

When I left last year, supplements did not play the biggest role anymore, which is great. Because food has become much more important to people, in general, and to athletes. But if I had gone into this job in 2006 with the view of no supplements, I may as well have taken my P45; it just wouldn't have worked. If you hadn't had plenty of life and professional experience, that's maybe the angle you would have taken, and understandably so. When I went in, we reviewed and looked at all supplements that were being used, aware that you weren't necessarily going to get the truth all of the time. But we got a really good overview of what was being used and why it was being used. Then back in 2007, I developed a sports supplement policy that viewed the appropriate use of supplements based on safety and efficacy. It was bought into mainly because the IRFU agreed to fund it. With professional players, we took the angle of we're protecting you here; we will take the hit if there's a problem. We have our traceability, and we have our line of testing, but if you step outside this, then it's on your head. So it took a good while to get buy-in to that. But it allowed the nutritionists (and there weren't that many around the country at that stage) to at least have the backing of the IRFU policy position on supplement use. All the professional clubs, in the four provinces of Ireland, were mandated to adhere to it. So I took the view, let's try to get supplement use regulated and managed and then work on building up the importance of and interest in food to be the cornerstone of nutrition support.

**Who are your mentors in life and why have they been mentors for you?**

**Ruth:** It's an interesting one. Family is important to me, especially in later years. I was one of four and we all went to boarding school. So I left home at the age of nine to go to school in Dublin having lived in the west of Ireland. As a result, I could not say that family were a huge influence during the early days. They were always there to support you of course, but maybe not on a day-to-day basis.

My professional colleagues and my friends (outside my profession) have been hugely important to me. Interestingly, I often would have reached out to people who were not in the profession; they were professional people, but they may be working in a different profession. I found that that was useful because they were not so close to either the issue, the problem or the situation and they could be more objective when looking towards a solution or a pathway to a solution.

I had some really strong dietetic colleagues who would have been great sounding boards. Within sports, I used my team of nutritionists hugely to be professional guides as well. I think it's a really good thing to have people around you that will support you and help you gain confidence and reassurance. It's really important and a challenge for us all to develop a system of available mentors.

This is something being considered by the SENR and I sit on a few committees of that register, where we're looking to develop a bank of people that are available for mentoring. It's all very well to say to people to go and get a mentor. But actually, where do all these new graduates find them? That was one of the reasons you set up your programme because there was that gap in doing it, and I think that's great. But we need to make sure it's wide and diverse in people's experience. I think your book editions here are adding to that as well.

**Yeah, if I'm honest, it's something that, I wasn't shocked by, but I kind of understood why SENR didn't have a mentorship programme.**

**Ruth:** I agree. SENR has grown in its development and also in its recognition as a quality competency register. I think the next step is looking at a framework for mentoring but of course, these things take time, and they also take money. They take people's willingness to be part of that. But it's something the registration committee will be driving for sure.

**What is a standout moment in your career so far?**

**Ruth:** The big one, for me, has been the development of the nutrition team. People might think, oh, it's the success that Irish Rugby has had, that's great and it's rewarding. Of course, they go and win a Grand Slam this year when I've just left but last year we had a triple crown and I've been part of two Grand Slams.

But if I reflect on it, it's developing the team of performance nutritionists that makes a performance difference and being in a position to be able to influence how services are provided. Emma Gardner is now the head of nutrition at the IRFU as a full-time position and she provides the services to the senior national team, as well as managing and developing the overall service. Pre-COVID, it was agreed that this position would be two positions; there would be a senior position with the senior national team and then there'd be a head of service who would concentrate on being the strategic lead for the nutrition service.

That took some hard grind to convince the performance director; the medical director was in support of this model. That was signed off and was ready to go in the summer of 2020 and then COVID hit, which was such a shame, because when you look at it, there's a head of physio, there's the head of what is called athletic performance or S&C, there's the head of medicine, and over those years developing nutrition as we did, it was time that there was a head of nutrition whose focus is the strategic direction and development of the nutrition service.

Unfortunately, that's not in place yet but Emma is on the case, and I just said, keep chipping away, keep chipping away. Because I do believe you need to be in the right place at the right time to be able to have the voice and influence practices and development of service. You need to be there; you don't need to be off in Paris during the Six Nations where you're missing those meetings. So being in a position to influence decision-makers is important. I think something important for practitioners to remember is that nutrition is only a small part of something bigger, and where it fits in and where, in fact, it is not going to add value. To be able to recognise that with athletes and programmes is important.

For example, I might have a passion for supporting a specific programme, but if there's no money to follow that, then forget it. I learned that very clearly in dietetics; focus on where there's going to be funding and where there's going to be interest. In the women's game, for example, at the moment, we have just got a full-time position in the women's pathway which was a result of a review of the Irish Women's programme. There is much more focus now on women's rugby worldwide.

This new position will involve supporting the women's pathway through professional clubs around the country. Some central contracts have been offered to players now which is progress. Putting your focus and energy into where you can see the next big thing is really important.

As I said success, of course, is great and they were just a great bunch to work with. We were a fairly cohesive management team, no more than what you can say of your own. We'd worked together for several years. I worked with four head coaches and they're all, as you know in your experience, very different. You have to learn how they want information and what they need to know, what they don't want to know or need to know. So reading the room is an important thing to learn.

So there is certainly more than one standout moment, but if I was to pick one, it would be about the development of the nutrition team for sure.

**Class. In terms of influential factors, why have you been so successful in your career to date? What is it that Ruth has that has allowed you to do what you've done?**

**Ruth:** Several things. As I've said, life and professional experience. You can't buy it; I think it's something that new practitioners may not have, and that's acceptable, of course. Everybody has to start and for them to understand that everything is not expected of them. If they try to do that, it may not be a good outcome. So life and professional experience help for sure.

Building relationships. Relationships are key in life, never mind in performance nutrition. Often in performance, you can be dealing with egos and strong individuals. You've got to find a way to build a relationship with those characters. For your good and keeping yourself in mind, what's best for you in your job, how can I manage these people? I've met plenty of people with whom I didn't necessarily agree with the way they were going about things, but you have to find a way to work with them which may require compromise on both sides. Communication is important; read the room, be able to listen and sit back and take it in and just work out where your best angle is in what you can bring. Knowing your stuff, of course, goes without saying and being willing to compromise. What I suppose a big thing is when you've done all that, keeping in mind how does performance nutrition add value? Where does it add value? We know it does, we're passionate about it, but not everybody else has got that same passion. We need to see it from their side, see it from their angle and we need to be able to convince decision-makers.

I had an example where I had to convince the head coach about the value of having a performance nutritionist who had the same line of accountability as other professional service providers in the programme. I talked about adding value. I said, look, I think it will, but you've got to see that it will. I said, here's the thing, I want you to trust me on this, give this a shot. If in six months, you think there's no value being added to your programme, we will review and rethink it. Anyway, he accepted this and within three months, he contacted me saying he wanted to extend her contract. One success story!

Equality of accountability for performance nutritionists was a big driver of mine in probably the last five years in my role. Historically nutritionists have a line of accountability through the S&C department. I believe there is no need for this. Performance nutrition has become a standalone profession and should be treated as such. When the opportunity arose, which was usually when there was a position vacancy, there was the opportunity to change that model. I had the support of the medical director, who used to engage with the head coach, and I wasn't at those meetings. That unsettled me a bit, but he said, look, you're too close to this and to be fair, he probably carried more influence than I did!

What I learned from that was to take advantage of whomever you need to help you to get the outcome you want. So whereas I would have preferred to have been in those meetings, I had to resign myself to a certain degree to say, right, well, they will get the job done and the outcome that I want at the end of it. So now in Irish Rugby, every lead nutritionist in the professional clubs is operationally accountable to the head coach and professionally accountable to the IRFU head of nutrition. This has created even better buy-in from senior management as the head coach has a responsibility to oversee and support the work of the performance nutritionist who is a member of their staff.

**That's superb. In terms of the opposite of wins and successes, what is a challenge that you've faced in your career that you're happy to share?**

**Ruth:** I think one that is ongoing for everybody is to educate decision-makers on what we do to add value to performance programmes. There are people out there who still feel we just make sure the lunch comes out on time. So we have to question ourselves as to why this is their impression and continue to educate and show them what we do. So perhaps changing our language a bit so they link what we do more with performance. To us, this probably feels like spin, but we need to use language that performance staff will regard as having a direct performance effect.

Another challenge is to remind yourself that you will not win every battle and decide which ones are worth fighting. I've had to make many of these decisions and there were plenty that I didn't win. But I needed to focus on the ones that I reckoned were the most important, certainly to the decision-makers.

I think for us to measure performance outcomes can be tricky. There are so many things that contribute to performance. Perhaps people link us with body composition as the only performance outcome of performance nutrition. However, in about the last five years, there's been an acceptance that while body composition will always remain an important element of an athlete's performance, there has been the realisation that over-focus on it can result in a negative association with food. This in turn may lead to disordered eating and/or Relative Energy Deficiency in Sport. So ensuring that athletes and performance staff understand that performance nutrition outcomes are much more than just body composition; understanding that proper nutrition supports health and resilience and performance optimisation through appropriate fuelling to delay fatigue and enhance recovery and optimal healing and recovery from injury, are important areas for practitioners to consider. We need to make sure that we develop performance outcomes to measure our true input to performance. We need to show that we can make a difference and why we need to be part of the athletes' programme.

Finally, having patience. Things take time to build. I was 16 years at the IRFU and there is still more to be developed. As far back as 2009 I presented my vision of the nutrition service to the organisation's main committee. I put together a paper about where I felt nutrition needed to go. This was the summary statement:

> A service model that is centrally contracted and consistent with other professionals within the organisation to allow for the responsibility of appointments, standards of conduct, performance, governance and ethics, as well as providing leadership to a team of practitioners with recognised qualifications and experience to deliver the services required.

That was in 2009 and it wasn't until 2022 that I could say, we were almost there. Nutrition staff are not all centrally contracted, they're contracted by their club, which is fine, provided your relationship is good. I still favour centrally contracted contracts, not because I wanted control; I wanted accountability.

**In terms of characteristics, what do you think people need to work in our industry? From that, do you have any recommendations for students entering the industry now? Then are there any topics that people aren't currently studying on courses, which could put them in a far better place when they graduate?**

**Ruth:** People need to be well qualified, for sure. I worked in the day when people who weren't qualified at all were working in this space. Thankfully, we're getting much better at that. So I think that people should get advice before they embark on undergraduate and postgraduate education. I've talked to many people who have done a course that isn't recognised, so potentially this means they've wasted their money and their time. So get advice about that. When starting, practitioners need to know their limitations and be willing to ask for help and guidance.

Attention to detail is one of my things; never underestimate it. Also, learn to understand the bigger picture of the field that you are working in. A particular characteristic is being able to relate to people, communicate well, and I'm sure many others have said this, but relationship building is crucial. That may not be easy; there'll be people you've come across that will knock you back. You've just got to try to find a way to make it a workable relationship. You don't have to be their friend but it costs nothing to be friendly. Adaptable, resilient, and able to relate all your actions to performance. I used to hesitate to say that because being from a dietetic background, for me, the fundamental is health. That's fine and it's great that we see that health is starting to play a much bigger role in sport now. Years ago, coaches didn't consider the importance of health and resilience so much. Now they see this as central to their athletes' well-being and subsequently their ability to perform.

So that's the characteristics. A recommendation to new practitioners coming in is to be smart when developing your CV. I have been on many interview panels, which I have enjoyed. It's been a fantastic opportunity. I like interviewing people and new graduates need to be smart; they need to tailor their CV to the position that they're applying for, not just put in a standard CV. Anyone can do that. Make yours stand out. Be careful, though, not to over-embellish it because the risk is you will get found out. Do your homework on the position you've applied for; know the organisation, speak to people and be as best prepared as you can be.

Don't fear failure. Everybody makes mistakes; we just need to recognise them and learn from them. As I've said many times, relate all actions to performance and health. I think a big one is to look for the simplest solutions. The more complicated something is, the less likely somebody's going to either follow it or be able to understand it for that matter. We deal with people with varying intellectual levels, so we need to be mindful of what they can understand.

Planning out your CPD path is important. Being a new graduate, you will think you need a lot of development, but there's no expectation you get there in the first year. I am a real advocate of the SENR, and I believe it will become an essential criterion for many jobs in the future.

It currently is an essential criterion in a lot of jobs in the UK. I think it is a really useful tool to assure you that you are competent to practise. This is a way in which we can capture the good people that are working in the world of sports. Walk before you can run and use people outside of your profession. I find that useful to help guide you and gain confidence. Forming interest groups of like-minded professionals which probably happens naturally. There are people that I would have as my go-to people, to bounce ideas around because it can be a lonely old world, especially if you're a sole trader, or a new practitioner just starting. So those would be my tips for newbies into the world of performance nutrition.

I was fortunate to come into the field of performance nutrition with a background in dietetics and the practical application of nutrition science is at the core of dietetic practice. This is a skill that I believe courses should always include as many students have not had the opportunity to embed the practical application of nutrition science. I'm pleased to see that many universities recognise the necessity of including that component and are now building this into the curriculum of their courses.

The approach to behavioural change has evolved so much over my years of practice. Back when I qualified, it was probably there in a different guise, but there wasn't as much focus on it. The psychology of eating I think is also a significant element that should be studied. I reckon we all agree that the mind plays a huge part in our nutrition habits.

**Yeah, it does. In five years, where are we going to be with nutrition?**

**Ruth:** Well, first of all, we're coming into the era where performance nutrition is recognised as a standalone discipline. I think that's important and a great place to be. I was around, as I say, in the day when people who weren't qualified in nutrition at all were working in the area. So that has changed greatly and that's great. I think, though, we do need to remember that performance nutrition is still a young discipline. We need to continue to show how we add value safely and effectively. In five years, I suspect nutrition will probably become more and more individualised based on emerging science. But I think we need to be mindful that there's still plenty of work to do in getting what we already know across to athletes and maybe the focus should be on how we do that. I mean, I left knowing that some players still believe that carbohydrate makes them fat. That's as much society telling them that as anything else because we've got to remember that athletes are people before they are athletes. They will be vulnerable, probably even more vulnerable, to society's messages than non-athletes are. So we need to continue to strive on how we get what we already know across to athletes as opposed to us or others, in fact, always looking for the next silver bullet.

I'm a real advocate that food is so much more than just fuel for the body. Sharing good food helps build relationships, build connections and that's healthy for our body and our mind. Food is such a powerful tool; you've seen it in your current work with your performance chef at Bristol Bears. We got a performance chef full time at the beginning of 2020, luckily, just before lockdown, and the difference that he has made has been huge. So much so that the old heads in the national team told me my job was done! But it has just heightened their interest in food and their enjoyment of food. We have a dining area that I was determined was not going to become a performance space; it has become a place where athletes and staff can enjoy good food and good company. We put up pictures of attractive food with the logo eat well, stay well and play well, as a reminder of the power of food. That's three years ago now and the interest in food has gained real momentum.

**That's brilliant. You mentioned that you flick through books. Is there one that stands out that you think was interesting recently; it doesn't have to be nutrition related?**

**Ruth:** I suppose on a performance front, one that I did find quite useful was the one by Ben Hunt-Davis and Harriet Beveridge – *Will It Make The Boat Go Faster?* I liked it because I'd be fairly goal orientated. It summarised at the beginning of the chapters about their goals and how to achieve them so I enjoyed that. I think the very title of it also marries in to the importance of added value. Is what you're doing adding value, will it make the boat go faster? If it doesn't, rethink your actions.

I read one on the recommendation of our medical director called *Being Mortal: Illness, Medicine and What Matters in the End* by Atul Gawande. It's not nutritionally related at all, but it's a really interesting take on how medicine and treatment of illness and disease have progressed over the years. Medics are trained to treat but they're not trained to teach people how to die and to respect that. Live a good life right to the end rather than focusing on a good death.

I read the memoir of Madeleine Albright, who was the first female US Secretary of State, and it just was a fascinating read about her as Madam Secretary, fleeing from a communist country with her diplomat family to the US as a young girl. For women, it shows the role you can play, but I think it was more than that. It was more than the fact that she was female, it was more about the facts of the world, of the battles and the relationships and the communication that you need to be prepared to take on the challenges you will face. I found that interesting.

**That's great. What key principles do you follow every day?**

**Ruth:** Get me out of bed at this stage! I strive to be happy. I strive to look at opportunities and take them now I'm retired from work, even though I'm still doing some education work within the profession. I think to work out what my purpose is now. It's interesting, James, because I've been asked, what is it you miss about work? The biggest thing I miss about work is people. It's not necessarily the work itself, but it's the people I've worked with. We've all worked with people that have been challenging, but generally speaking, the supportive people will outweigh those. I used to come back home up here in the north, from work with the IRFU, which is full on and full of people, and the nicest thing I wanted to do was put my feet up, with a glass of wine and watch TV, and I was happy enough to do that. But now that I don't have all those people around me, I do miss them.

Every day I work at connections, making connections, reconnecting with people that I perhaps have lost connection with, through working away from home for so long. Trying to be a good person and being kind too. We don't always do those things all of the time but we should strive for it. I'm a bit of a list person, probably more operationally on what I want to get done. It's satisfying to tick them off!

So I think to be happy and to look at opportunities and take them when you can. There are people in such hard situations that you should count your blessings for what you've got. I still have a way to go in my so-called retirement plan. It certainly wasn't the first year of retirement that I planned because of my new springer spaniel pup who has had two surgeries in her first year. But that sort of taught me a few things, and I plan that my next year will be different. I want to continue to travel; I have a camper van and the plan is for me and my dog to be off on our travels. Some of the things I had in my mind for my first retirement year were unrealistic and that maybe isn't a bad thing to realise. I do think I'm lucky to be in this situation and I plan to make the most of it.

**Okay, Ruth, finally then, to probably summarise our interview and to give those that read this book some concluding thoughts and remarks: in your eyes, in your experience, in all of the interview panels you've sat on, with all of the practitioners that you've seen go on to have great careers, what is it that makes those performance nutritionists successful in their careers?**

**Ruth:** Okay, well, top of my list would be knowledge and the ability to translate that into practice. That is easier said than done. New graduates will come out with all the theory and it's a lifelong learning curve that you need to constantly navigate. Work out what works and what doesn't work. For sure, communication, relationships, respect, and having an open mind are all really important characteristics that somebody needs to work on, not only in this space but in lots of others.

In your practice, I think you need to decide what is negotiable and what is not; stick to your professional principles. But find a way to communicate that is not going to offend people or compromise your development. But stick with your principles. You're educated to a level that merits the respect and trust of your professional gut, I suppose. We need to find the simplest solutions. There's so much noise in the nutrition world that it's easy to get sort of swept up in it and forget that often the simplest solutions work best.

Finally, be aware of where you as a performance nutritionist fit into the bigger picture of your work environment. Be able to see where you get the biggest gains and be also able to see where nutrition isn't going to add anything to a certain situation and be honest with that. Being confident to do that takes time.

**Yeah. Superb. That's outstanding. What an interview!**

## JAMES'S THOUGHTS

Ruth is the reason Irish rugby has performance nutritionists embedded in most, if not all rugby teams at club level. It was so interesting to hear how Ruth was part of the original intake of BDA accredited dietitians back in 1994.

Ruth speaks eloquently about the importance of life, professional experience and building relationships. These all come with practice and the more you do the better you become.

I call this craft knowledge. It is the knowledge you develop from being in the trenches, with the athletes, making mistakes and learning from them!

A gem which you may have missed in this chapter is the part where you remind yourself that you will not win every battle and you need to decide which ones are worth fighting. I have had my fair share of these during my career!

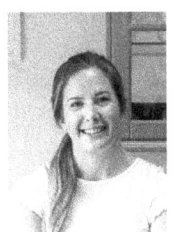

## CHAPTER 6:
## LAUREN DELANY

Lauren is a professional rugby union player for Sale Sharks Rugby Club and holds the role of lead performance nutritionist at the club for the women's team. She is also the nutritionist with the men's first team and academy with Sale Sharks. Lauren is also internationally capped, having represented Ireland rugby for the last five years.

Lauren has an MSc in sport and exercise nutrition from Loughborough University and is currently studying her PhD at Leeds Beckett University in optimising body composition in professional rugby players through sports nutrition intervention and behavioural science.

Lauren and I crossed paths in the world of rugby. Where else, hey!! We have also met in person at a few conferences and always enjoyed talking all things rugby, nutrition and research.

You can follow Lauren on:
Twitter @LaurenVeronaD
Instagram @laurenveronanutrition

**For those that don't know who you are, who are you and what are you currently doing?**

**Lauren:** I kind of describe my life as wearing three different hats professionally, but I obviously have my personal life as well. I suppose the first hat that I wear is that I'm a performance nutritionist with the English Gallagher Premiership rugby union team, Sale Sharks, where I work with the men's team and the men's academy and I've been there for one season. I have previously spent two years in rugby league working with the Super League's Leeds Rhinos men's first team who got to the grand final last season. Then previous to that, I spent seven years with the English Institute of Sport (EIS), working with a range of different sports. The first two years, I was a bit of a jigsaw puzzle between GB Badminton, British Skeleton, I did some time with British Taekwondo, British Swimming and then I got the opportunity to join British Cycling for five years. That was supporting the team in the lead-up to the Rio 2016 Olympic and Paralympic Games and then Tokyo 2020 as well. I suppose within that role, I was the sprint specialist working with track sprint, the different BMX squads and then working with the whole of the Paralympic programme as well. That's the first hat I wear. The second hat is that I'm studying for my PhD in the Carnegie Applied Rugby Research group at Leeds Beckett University; I'm heading into my third year now and I'm all about exploring how we help players optimise their body mass and body composition through behaviour change science. The final cap that I wear professionally or semi-professionally is that I'm an international rugby union player with 22 senior caps for Ireland. I have been part of the squad for five years now. I play my domestic rugby as the co-captain of Sale Sharks women's team playing in the Premier 15s in England in the top flight so a few hats and a lot of things to juggle.

**What cap do you prefer to wear?**

**Lauren:** I think right now in my life the priority overall is probably my own personal rugby because it's so short-lived; it could end tomorrow and be gone. It can end next week whereas I can always finish my PhD. I can always spend years being a nutritionist in the future. I can explore different routes but being an international rugby player and playing at the top level is so short-lived, and for me, it's almost a second wind of my athletic career. I played basketball for 15 years and I only started playing rugby at 25. So I feel like it's a once in a lifetime opportunity. If I don't put everything into it right now then I could regret it in the future.

**Yeah, nice. I was going to ask that, have you always played rugby? But yeah, evidently not. So you've always been an athlete growing up? Were you international standard in basketball as well?**

**Lauren:** Yeah, under age I played internationally at European championships and the younger age groups, but unfortunately, we lost all funding in Ireland for the senior teams when I think I was 17 or 18 at the time, or maybe even 19, I think when I'd done my Leaving Certificate (equivalent to A levels), so there weren't actually any senior teams to even play for; you could only play for the national league in Ireland.

**You mentioned earlier that the EIS was some of your first exposure into nutrition. Did you study nutrition as an undergrad? Or was it more of a conventional sports science and then you kind of found your way into nutrition?**

**Lauren:** So I was one of those weirdos who people hated back in school at 15/16. You'd go and see the guidance counsellor and you discuss all your options. You do all these tests. I kind of knew before even going in there that I wanted to get into nutrition. I wanted to probably work in sports as well because I played basketball and I loved it. I suppose all the calculations and everything they did, they kind of said, well, look, your best route is going down the dietetics route and becoming a dietitian. Sports science from what I remember wasn't very big in Ireland back then in terms of degrees and courses. It probably didn't even come up as an option for me. I did my undergraduate in human nutrition and dietetics jointly between the University of Dublin, Trinity College and the Technological University of Dublin as well. So that was four and a half years. So I did nutrition and dietetics and qualified as a dietitian. Then 10 years ago now I came over to England to do my master's at Loughborough University in sport and exercise nutrition.

**When you started your role at the EIS, what was your favourite sport to do the nutrition support with?**

**Lauren:** Well, when I started off, it was just British Badminton two days a week. Over the course of two years, I built up an extra day here, an extra day there, kind of a short-term role here, there and everywhere. I suppose the most consistent role there was British Badminton; I really enjoyed that experience. For me, the standout one was definitely the initial months I worked with British Skeleton. It was a winter sport and over those two years, I hadn't worked with any other winter sports. It was so niche; it was so different to anything that I had experienced before. In terms of their performance demands, they're essentially sprinting for a few seconds and then they're lying on a sled going headfirst in the freezing cold winter down a bobsled track. When I was thinking back about the questions you were asking for this book, this was probably one of my first exposures in terms of body weight and body composition and whether it's important or whether it's not important. If you're sprinting for three seconds, does fat mass really matter? Is it more important to be as heavy as possible? But there was a max weight that you could be between your body weight and the sled as well. So you were working within some constraints. But it was just such a crazy sport, really challenging, but a really good time as well and great athletes to work with. So I loved that in the early days.

**Just for my education here, I imagine that weight on the sled would result in momentum after time but only so much weight. So were there ever acute weight loss strategies that these athletes would try and follow to be as strong and powerful as possible but then an hour or a day before they try and drop maybe three kilos to be a little bit lighter?**

**Lauren:** No, because if you were lighter, you put more weight on the sled. So there was that max weight that whether you hit it with your body weight or with the sled was that weight, so there was never a need to do that. It was almost always the question of well, I might as well be that maximum weight, regardless of what it looks like. I might as well have that full momentum from me, as opposed to the sled. There were loads of challenging questions: is there a point in even assessing body comp? In those early days, you know yourself, I definitely didn't have the confidence to be able to step back and say no, or really establish whether it was important or not.

**Who were or are some of your biggest mentors in life right now? And why are they important for you?**

**Lauren:** So thinking back over the years, in terms of who have been the mentors, there's almost different types of mentors in your life. I think some of those early years in terms of my dietetics degree, the one lecturer, one person that always stood out was Dr Claire Corish. She was a senior lecturer, head of the course, but also a bit of a distant relative to me as well so I kind of knew of her anyway. She's always the one that stood out in terms of that inspirational female figure who always spoke so well and was really highly regarded. You could always have a conversation with her. She was interested a little bit in that sports nutrition side as well. I think I was the only person in my course at the time that was interested in sports nutrition, rather than the medical route of dietetics. So we always had those kinds of conversations. She definitely stands out as one of those in the past. She's still interested in my career today and always asks questions and is supportive on social media. She's a big advocate for my rugby as well. In more recent years my PhD supervisors Prof Susan Backhouse and Prof Ben Jones are huge mentors for me. They're such inspirational figures in academia and professional sport. They're really supportive but also encouraging and know how and when to challenge me to get the best from me.

In terms of probably the more stereotypical mentors or line managers that I had in the English Institute of Sport, there were many in the early days. Kevin Currell and Mike Naylor were the obvious ones, in probably a different role in that I only saw them once a month, once every few months; they were external to the jobs I was doing. They were always brilliant in terms of encouragement, having that balance between encouragement and challenge and really kind of testing how I was going. For me, the one that always stands out, and probably still to this day, is Kathryn Brown. Again, a line manager, but a unique situation, which you've probably experienced at the Football Association, but it doesn't happen very often, two full-time practitioners working within the same sport, on the desk beside each other.

That was a brilliant experience. I owe a lot of what I know and how I practise today to Kathryn. She was an unbelievable practitioner with a ton of experience, very different personality to me, but I think we complemented each other really well. She knew how to balance that mentoring and line managing knowing that she comes to life with very different kind of characteristics. She was probably the best and still is to this day in terms of balance between supporting me as a practitioner, technically, but also kind of personally as well, like taking the whole me into account. If there were some days that I was really struggling, whether it's professionally or personally, she'd always be there. She'd always be someone that would listen. It had that nice balance in particular. Like I said, she's still a dear friend, and definitely a mentor today.

I suppose, where I am at the minute and the more I think about who would be my mentors today, I almost see them as peer mentors at the minute. So those who are probably at the same level in different ways, one of my good friends, Hannah Crowley, would probably be a good mentor in terms of the practitioner side. She's a sport and sport rehab therapist, but also an S&C coach. She works for British Cycling but she's great in terms of, "You know, I'm dealing with this athlete in this situation at the minute, like what would you do? How would you go about that?" She is always one of those people that gives brilliant advice.

The other peer mentor I have at the minute would be in the PhD side and a PhD student and a lecturer now, she's just finished a PhD, Lucy Chesson. Because she's two, three years ahead of me, in terms of the PhD journey, she just has this wealth of knowledge in terms of the research methodology I'm using, as well as the little things in the day-to-day life of a PhD student, but again, has that lovely balance of reminding me that I'm human; if I need a break, go for it. She reminds me that this isn't the be-all and end-all, just that lovely balance between the personal and professional mentor in particular. I have some rugby mentors, but we don't need to go into them as well.

**You've got three hats that you wear and you've also had some amazing experiences with the EIS as you mentioned, Olympic Games, winter and summer sports. Is there a standout moment in your career to date? From either one of the hats or one from each hat?**

**Lauren:** I could definitely do one from each hat. This is a really difficult question to answer and think of what has been a standout moment. For me, there are different types of standout moments. I can't not talk about when I got that first role with British Cycling, the most successful Olympic and Paralympic sport in the country for the last three, four Olympics cycles. That has to be a standout getting that role, working full time in one sport as a nutritionist for the first time as well. In those early days, I never really thought it would be possible to work full time within one role. It has to be one of those standout periods of time working with them. It was also one of the most challenging times of my life over those few years, in terms of the media, in terms of all the investigations that have gone on in terms of everything, from claims of sexism, to bullying, to anti-doping, to everything that went on. That's equally standout in terms of the most challenging and things you never expected to happen.

In terms of the PhD, my first study has been interviewing rugby league players on their lived experiences of body composition, assessment and exploring some of the enablers and barriers that they experienced to manage their body composition and body mass. A standout interview for me was with a player where we were exploring body composition, but also exploring all the in-depth levels of this player's childhood, their experiences and their upbringing and how all of this, all these parts of their journey and their identity, influence how they view their body, how they eat the food, whether they weigh themselves or not. There was this one athlete who highlighted some sad traumas in their childhood, which was a really, really challenging interview that was over 90 minutes. There were floods of tears afterwards, it was just such a sad interview. Really difficult one but again, it stands out for me in highlighting that we're not just talking about a person's body weight and what they're eating and doing today. We're exploring as practitioners, as researchers, their entire life and their upbringing and their childhood. For us not to explore that with players in as much depth with athletes as possible, I think is almost naive.

In terms of my rugby career, a stereotypical standout moment was my first cap for Ireland, but probably the one that stands out for me and still gives me goosebumps today was in my second cap for Ireland. We played at Twickenham, in front of 10,000 people straight after the men's game. I think they were playing Australia at the time, and I scored my first try for Ireland and still to this day I get goosebumps thinking about it. That has to be a standout moment in front of 10,000 people. My whole family, my extended family, were there as well. I don't think I've ever experienced anything like that before.

**And were they there at the end where you scored the try?**

**Lauren:** They actually were; they were at the end in the corner.

**Nutritionists doing one to ones or having an unbelievably close relationship with the psychologist at the club, how important is that considering what you've just said?**

**Lauren:** It's so important. Working alongside a sports psychologist in the previous roles has been invaluable and has helped me to manage some of the biggest challenges in nutrition. Unbelievably important. Probably in more recent years in rugby, when there hasn't been psychology support available, it's probably highlighted to me even more the value of that. If I could have every one-to-one conversation with the psychologist beside me, not only would we be providing a better and more holistic support service to players but I would also be a better practitioner too.

**Interesting. My next question here is related to the body composition assessment. You're doing some really interesting research in this space now. There's also a lot of talk across institutes on social media around, should we even be doing body compositions anymore within clubs? What's your view on that?**

**Lauren:** Oh, that's a challenge. I'm just writing my practical recommendations on my paper so I can't give too much away. I think in terms of body composition assessment, I don't think we can completely move away and get rid of it completely. We'd be naive and stupid to say we should never do it again. I think there must be a more player-centred focus with assessing. It has to be voluntary; I think there has to be consent involved with it and I think it has to be done in a more sensitive way than we have done in the past. There is value to it but there is a way it has almost gotten a bit out of control in terms of why we're assessing, how we're assessing, how we're feeding it back and how much priority and importance we're placing on the result, in comparison to other elements of performance. So I still think there's a role for it in sport, just that us as practitioners as well as culturally, I think we can do it a lot better and have the player involved. Essentially, if the player refuses, there's a lot to explore there, but it's their body and I think they should be within their rights to not be assessed.

**I've spoken about this numerous times with different practitioners and on podcasts and what we moved away from with the Lionesses was doing skinfold assessment in isolation. So we would track skinfolds because that was the only method we could do; we would take away any reporting of body fat percentage, because we didn't want to put it on there. We would even take away the numbers on the graphs so they didn't know whether they were 70mm, 90mm, 56mm, etc. We would then track it alongside counter movement jump, or alongside speed, or alongside hamstring strength, or alongside the 1k time trial. What we were trying to get across to the girls and I've used this really successfully at Bristol Bears is body composition is not a fat measurement; body composition is a functional mass assessment. Are you the most functional athlete you can be in your position right now? What you then find is that, normally the guys that are carrying quite a bit of extra mms or fat mass are the ones that are quite slow on a 1k time trial; you can show them that on the graph. You can say, look, there's a really strong correlation here of those that have lower total mms are the ones that are actually fitter.**

**So my aim with you as an individual is I'm trying to move you into the green zone. The way that we can do that is to improve your body composition. So that conversation I found to be so much more successful because not once did I measure or mention body fat percentage, fat mass, skinfold**

thickness; it's all about, I'm trying to get you to be more explosive. I'm trying to be able to get you to jump higher in lineouts, that's what I'm trying to get you to do. I shared that with Graeme at the recent BDA Sport Nutrition event. It was really interesting to hear other people's thoughts on that. Because in my mind, it's a no-brainer. An absolute no-brainer, but it's a conversation for another day.

**What do you think has been one of the most influential factors as to why you've been, I say this word, successful? Because when you define successful in the dictionary, it's the accomplishment or an achievement of a goal. So that doesn't mean that you're the best nutritionist in the world. It doesn't mean that I am, it doesn't mean that Louise Burke is, but why do you think you've got to where you have in your career? What is it that you've got that maybe some of the other students that are coming through may be able to learn or pick up from?**

**Lauren:** For me, it's all about being a people person and building relationships. In terms of the interviews that I've been involved with, in terms of interviewing for other roles and jobs, it's rarely the technical side of nutrition. It's normally what's their character like? Will they get on with people? Will they work well as part of a team? How have they put themselves across? Do we think they're going to hit the ground running? They're the more important questions rather than did they know the amount of protein that that athlete should have at this point in time. I know for me, that's definitely one of my biggest strengths in terms of building relationships with people, being comfortable having conversations with athletes that have nothing to do with nutrition, that have nothing to do with food, that's about their day to day and the challenges that they face and some of the great things going on in their life.

I suppose on one side of it, that's probably a little bit of my kind of personality, my character from that. But it's certainly something that I have put a lot of time, effort and work into. I've always made a huge effort, no matter who I'm talking to, whether I know them or not, to get to know them, to talk to them, to give them my full time and my full attention. With nutrition at the end of the day, the majority of what we do is advise people, and whether they take on that advice or not, there has to be an underlying level of a relationship and of trust and of understanding for them to go away and take that advice and implement it. So for me, I think in all parts of the three different hats that I wear, a lot of it is that ability to build relationships, whether that's really quickly in short periods of time or over a longer time and in sports and try to get to know people. I feel like that's probably the most standout one that I come back to anyway.

**What's been the biggest challenge of your career today?**

**Lauren:** So I chose two but I feel like they're very different routes. And so I'm gonna go through both of them.

I think one's probably a little bit more stereotypical in terms of the practitioner role. Again speaking of body composition and probably weight loss in particular, I'd say in every sport that I've been involved with, there has been one, maybe two athletes that no matter what you try, no matter what you do, you can't help them to lose weight. I was thinking through this. I literally have an example of one athlete in every single sport that was just known as this conundrum. When I think back on each of those athletes, that conundrum has progressed to be a smaller conundrum as the years go on. In those early days, you'd give them this really strict meal plan, 10 years ago, and you have no idea why they wouldn't follow it. You've no idea whether they did or didn't follow it and they couldn't lose weight. There was obviously a lot more going on behind the scenes.

I'll never forget this one athlete and they ended up being dropped from the programme and one of the reasons was due to their body weight. This was a major element that they couldn't lose the weight that they needed. I remember years later, talking to this athlete and them saying to me, "You had no idea what was going on behind the scenes"; nobody did. This person was struggling with addiction, with things not food related; they were struggling with pretty major mental health issues as well. They said to me, regardless of what you were doing, you had the best intentions. But there were certain elements of that, that had nothing to do with food. That always stands out to me as being a real moment where I realised it's not all about food, it's not all about a meal plan or what you give to an athlete, it's about what else is going on in their life.

There was another athlete, where I knew a lot more of what was going on. There were pretty major family illnesses going on with this athlete. Again, I'd say about two or three years with this athlete trying to get them to get to a certain weight and it was within a sport where weight and mass, in particular, were extremely important. That was the first time I had a joint meeting with a psychologist between me, the psych and the athlete. For those first three meetings that we had, they were absolutely nothing related to food, nothing related to nutrition, but all about how they process the world, the things that are going on behind the scenes and how very likely they're using food and other things as potentially coping mechanisms for dealing or not being able to deal with emotions and other situations that were going on. For me, those three years were unbelievably challenging.

That was a real turning point for me in terms of working with athletes in general and all those years of really challenging situations where you can't help them to lose weight, don't know what's going on. Is it my meal plan, maybe it is? Maybe I'm doing something wrong? Really questioning everything and probably over the years coming to that realisation that there's more going on in the background.

The other big challenge within my career was actually in the first season I got on the Irish team, with unbelievable time constraints and demands. In terms of leading into a Six Nations every weekend from Friday to Sunday, you'd be away on a training camp, then you come back Monday morning, you'd be in work Monday to Friday, and then Friday afternoon, you'd be gone again. I suppose the biggest challenge for that was, in your career and what you're working on day to day, I had to leave at five, there was no option not to, every evening was gone with training. I didn't have evenings, I didn't have weekends to catch up on any work. In terms of trying to balance, the work-life balance was unbelievably challenging for those few months in that first squad. It really forced me to be unbelievably time efficient and organised more than I ever had been. Because I only had that set amount of time during the week. I had no leeway. I had no other spare time to make up for it. In terms of work-life balance that was probably the most challenging experience in my career so far.

**What characteristics do you think people need to work in nutrition? You touched on a little bit of this earlier with the personality that an individual needs, someone that can fit into a group as well as work with other team members, but are there any other things that you would add into that if you're on an interview panel? What would make a candidate stand out?**

**Lauren:** I think the first one has to be, you've got to be able to translate the science into food. It's got to be the most simple thing that you've got to be able to do as a practitioner and within that, be able to translate advice into different environments, different sports and with different situations. That's an unbelievably important one. Being a people person and relationship building, as I mentioned, is definitely another one.

The ones that are a bit more difficult maybe to assess in an interview, for example, are probably to do with problem solving in particular; for example if something goes wrong with the food at a major event, how do you problem solve? A prime example of that I could give was, there was a World Cup event locally with teams staying at a hotel around the corner from the National Cycling Centre in England, literally, you could walk there, we went through the menus with the chefs and catering manager. We planned everything well in advance. We talked to the chefs and planned everything. On that first day, everything went wrong; it was absolutely awful. The food was terrible, it was undercooked, it was all coming out late, there was too little of it, the cutlery was dirty, everything that could have gone wrong. There were people getting ill as well. For us, it was all about that problem solving, being there on the ground, trying to find solutions to some of those little things, working with the staff, being able to problem solve, maybe not in terms of food and nutrition, but in terms of just the day-to-day stuff it's unbelievably important. Then, you can't move away from your ability to work within high pressure environments. When push comes to shove, it's really stressful and things do go wrong, how do you react, and your ability to stay calm, to problem solve, to manage some of those situations is really important, especially, not only in Olympic and Paralympic sports where it's one event, or leads into one event, but some of the most stressful environments have been those holding camps in the lead-in to Olympic and Paralympic Games where it could be something as small as there's no bread with this meal because we've run out, and you've got to find solutions. But there's a lot of pressure that goes on in those environments. You've got to be able to deal with it; you've got to be able to deal with the highs and lows of sports.

Yeah, I agree with that. One thing that I would add is, because I'm experiencing it right now, Bristol Bears are bottom of the league. When things are going well, and you're in the top four and it's all hunky dory, it's sunshine and rainbows. But when you're bottom of the league, it's interesting to see how characters may change. One thing that I've tried to maintain myself is that I'm a glass half full person all the time. It doesn't matter how bad it is. Even when I lost my father four years ago: what do I do, I can't control it. Let's crack on. That's something that I always try and maintain. It's interesting because I wasn't in the club for about three weeks leading into Christmas and the players were asking where is he? He's normally that energy and that character that we come and see every day. It was amazing, because I was thinking that they're not even coming to see me to ask me about nutrition, they just want to come and see me for a bit of a pickup. Being a good traveller with a team is important, someone who is a good person on camp with players. I think that's something that practitioners should always remember as well because when the going gets tough and fingers start pointing, you've really got to show your actual character and try and maintain your integrity.

So for a younger self or aspiring students trying to enter the industry now, our industry I think is changing a lot. When I started studying years ago, behaviour change wasn't even a topic. You've then got this, the applied nature of sports nutrition, getting out of the lab and actually being a person in a club. Now we've got the wonderful world of AI technology and things like Hexis. So a student starting now, what is your advice to that student for them to come and get a career in nutrition?

**Lauren:** I have placement students at the minute so I think about this a lot. I think the first thing that always stands out for me, and the thing that I always advise them, is that never assume that an athlete is convinced of the benefits of nutrition, that they'll buy in automatically, because students always think, they're an athlete and of course, why wouldn't all athletes do everything they need to improve performance? I thought like that coming out of my master's as well. Coming into my first role, I couldn't understand why I'm the expert, I'm giving them all this information to improve their performance, why aren't they following it? I think, again, it's just this assumption that all of this knowledge and all of this research that of course, athletes will do it, but they don't, of course they don't, there's got to be a lot of convincing involved. You have to get good at convincing as well. I think that's the first one, that you just can't assume that they're going to follow what you advise or that they're even going to be interested in it.

I'm not long with Sale Sharks, but there's a few athletes who have literally in those first few weeks come up to me and said no offence, it's nothing to do with you, it's nothing to do with you personally, it's just, I'm not into this nutrition thing. I'm just not interested. So you probably don't need to talk to me kind of straightaway. They're just not interested. For me it's allowing that and to say, that's absolutely fine, let's talk about something else and I'll try build a relationship a different way. Nine times out of 10 we will end up talking food and nutrition a few months down the line.

But again, if I was a master's student coming out of university 10 years ago, that would have completely taken me aback; I would have thought it my job to convince someone of the absolute opposite. So that's probably a big one. The other one again comes back to a bit of my PhD and our conversation earlier, but don't let weight loss, weight gain, body composition, be the sole purpose, or the sole focus or the first focus of your support.

There are many, many other elements of nutrition that are even more valuable. But it tends to be because body weight and composition are numbers and we like to evaluate performance based on numbers and not subjective data. It's objectively measured so it seems to be the first thing that everyone is interested in jumping on. Don't let that be the first thing; try and focus on all the other great elements of nutrition that can improve performance. Just don't just let that be the sole focus.

**So true. Even those quick wins of identifying that someone's probably not eating enough on the day of the game and bringing in an extra 50-60 grams of carbs at breakfast, that could be the only thing that you speak to them about for three weeks.**

**Are there any areas that you didn't learn on your course? Which now that you're a player, in particular, a PhD student, as well as a nutritionist, you wish that you had learned and studied a little bit in more detail on your course and that you've had to almost pick up as a practitioner?**

**Lauren:** Yeah, you've already highlighted that there; the entire element of behaviour change and motivational interviewing is massive. I'd probably highlight that more in terms of my master's. There was very little in terms of: you've got an athlete in front of you, how do you conduct an interview? How do you get all the information out of them? How do you build that relationship in the space of 20 minutes? How do you then give advice, create goals, get them to go away and do something about it, but while they might not want to change? In saying that, in the dietetics degree we actually did quite a lot of that. It is a professional degree in terms of allied health professionals so we actually do modules on psychology, on behaviour change, we actually have exams in terms of how you conduct an interview, you get judged on your level of motivational interviewing, you get videoed, you get feedback on that interview. In terms of the dietetics degree there was quite a lot, but in terms of doing a master's and a bit more sports science focus there wasn't any of that.

It really highlighted during my master's, that those who came from a dietetics background could qualify and go into a sports role tomorrow in comparison to those from a sports science background who just needed to grow and develop those soft skills a bit more. The other side, which is leading on from what we've just said, it's almost probably not learning more but helping young practitioners to understand how to prove their impact outside of the numbers of weight. So proving your value and your worth, the potential impacts that you can have, maybe not to winning a game, but to having a player who's better fuelled, and potentially using more qualitative quotes and other elements to prove impact in terms of that feedback from those players.

Oh, well, the player said they felt a lot better in the game, that they felt they have more energy during those last 10 minutes, using that as elements to prove impact in terms of some of your nutrition as opposed to just the basic numbers, which sometimes, if you're just focusing on body weight, or body composition, or some other elements, you can lose a lot of that other stuff. I still struggle and find that really, really challenging to this day, but I think we can do a lot more of the practitioner side of that in universities.

**Is there a motivational interviewing course that is aimed at dietitians or nutritionists working in sport?**

**Lauren:** I think the BDA provide some motivational interviewing and courses. I think they're pretty meaty and expensive. I've seen one or two of them. But outside of that, I haven't seen it from a nutrition perspective. I would assume from a psychology perspective, there would be versions of that. But yeah, I haven't heard of many of those.

**So where do you think the future of nutrition will be in five years' time? There's a lot going on right now and it moves quickly. One thing that stands out for me is the AI technology; you can ask what is a ketogenic diet, and all of a sudden you've got a paragraph on it. So that's happened since November 2022. Where do you think we're gonna be in five years in the nutrition space?**

**Lauren:** I mean, you've already highlighted with the likes of Hexis, the technology side of automated nutrition plans and food plans and support through technology. I think that's certainly going to blow up over the next five years. It kind of links in with that side of increased autonomy and independence for athletes, that they're in control of things a lot more, rather than relying on others; it gives them a lot more autonomy with that. So I think that's the next five to 10 years, that's the way it's going.

**Have you read any books recently that you've really enjoyed? It doesn't have to be nutrition, it can be anything. Is there anything that you like? One for me that stands out is *Atomic Habits by James Clear*, and *Deep Work by Cal Newport*. So what are you reading?**

**Lauren:** I was thinking about *Atomic Habits*. I love that book, in terms of behaviour change, and a different way of viewing it. The book I'm reading at the minute is the memoir of Kellie Harrington, the Irish boxer who won gold at Tokyo. I just loved it, because it talks about her childhood, run-ins with the police, experimenting with drugs and doing all these things at a young age and then boxing was the change for her which changed her life. She talks a little bit about her food journey as well, getting to work with a nutritionist. I love autobiographies, sports autobiographies and seeing where athletes come from and all the different backgrounds that there are, how athletes can progress through different life situations.

**Are there any key principles that you follow every day to keep you on the straight and narrow?**

**Lauren:** Write a to-do list every day at the start of the day; that is key one for me, because it gives me a plan for the day, and I love ticking stuff off as well.

This one is a challenge, but I try my best: any athlete interactions or any notes I need to write up at work, I try and write them up by the end of the day before I leave. Because, honestly, you get a few days later and you've hardly any idea of what the notes on the page actually meant, so trying to write athlete notes up by the end of the day. They would probably be the two key ones.

**Finally, in your mind and your experience and what you've seen, a brief answer as to what makes a successful performance nutritionist.**

**Lauren:** I would say a practitioner who has experience in a range of different environments, that has the ability to build relationships quickly. That they're comfortable being uncomfortable and in high pressure environments.

## JAMES'S THOUGHTS

Lauren is a fine example of practise what you preach! A nutritionist working in professional sport, a PhD student working in professional sport and finally a professional athlete, of course, in professional sport!

If there is one practitioner who is right on the heartbeat of what the athlete wants and what the athlete needs, then it's Lauren!

It was nice to hear Lauren talk about the importance of body composition in sport and importantly how it needs to be more player-centred. I'm confident that my functional mass project at Bristol Bears is my best ever integration of body composition assessment into the athletic performance department.

Lauren highlights again the importance of building better relationships and also how understanding behaviour change is going to be important, especially for practitioners moving forward as we continue to see the impacts of AI technology.

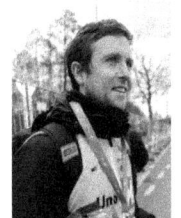

## CHAPTER 7:
# JAMES MORAN

James is the head of nutrition at Uno-X Pro Cycling Team. He has previously worked for INEOS Grenadiers, British Cycling and the English Institute of Sport. He has experience in both being a clinical dietitian and performance nutrition.

James and I have both studied at Liverpool John Moores University. James completed his MSc at LJMU before embarking on his career in professional sport. He has a wealth of experience in both Olympic teams and endurance cycling.

He is open to sharing some of the applied performance nutrition strategies he implements with his athletes on his Twitter account.

You can follow James on:
Twitter @JamesEPMoran

**For those that don't know who you are, and kind of what you're about, what is your background? And where did it all start with yourself?**

**James Moran:** Yeah, so I had a bit of a long journey to being a performance nutritionist. So originally when I was doing my A levels back in 2001, I wanted to be a physio; that is what I thought I wanted to be. I knew I wanted to be involved in sport and health and medicine. I was aware of people who were physios in football clubs and things like that. So that was kind of at the back of my mind. I thought, yeah, that'd be a cool career. I did PE as an A level, didn't think anything of it, it was my favourite subject. Then when it came to applying for uni, they said you needed chemistry or biology to do physio. Okay. So then I applied to do a sports science degree. There weren't that many programmes at the time but they were becoming more popular and it seemed to cover the things that I was interested in: physiology and biology and everything to do with sport and performance. So I went off on my way to Sheffield Hallam as a cocky 18-year-old lad from Oldham, to do a sports science degree. It was in the nutrition modules that we did, one of our tutors was Nigel Mitchell who was a dietitian, and he was working with British Cycling. At the time, it was when Olympic funding was coming, he used to come in his Great Britain kit and he was telling us all these stories about cycling and stuff and how he was working in different sports.

It was those modules that kind of really resonated with me. I did a nutrition-based dissertation looking at hydration and sodium. So when it came towards the end of finishing my degree, I thought, yeah, well, I want to work in nutrition, but there wasn't really a career path to being a sports nutritionist at that time as such. So I kind of finished, I wanted to travel and go to Australia and I was playing amateur rugby league at the time. So I saved for a year and went to Australia, did a bit of backpacking and played some amateur rugby league over there. Then when I came back, I thought I really wanted to try and get into this nutrition line of work. So I applied to do the postgraduate diploma in nutrition and dietetics at University of Chester and Leeds Beckett University to train to be a dietitian. I was doing jobs in call centres, working on building sites, did a bit of work as a gym instructor whilst trying to get on to being a dietitian. This job cropped up in my local hospital to be an assistant dietitian. So I thought this would be great because part time I could work as a gym instructor a few days a week, do the dietetic assistant job and get on the course and I'd become a dietitian really quick. So that happened in 2005. Then I applied to get on the dietitian training, but didn't get on. I got rejected because I got a 2.2 in my undergrad. I didn't have a science A level; they said they acknowledged that I had some experience as an assistant dietitian but said, maybe apply again. So I applied the year after and didn't get on. I thought what more do I need to do? So they said, if you study some modules in public health nutrition that you have to pay for yourself, we'll maybe consider you the year after but we can't guarantee it; there's a lot of strong academic applicants out there. So I did a third year working as an assistant dietitian and doing other part-time jobs. I kind of thought if it doesn't happen this year, I need to look at a different career. Maybe it's something telling me being a dietitian isn't going to work. So I was looking at cardiac/respiratory physiology training schemes in the NHS and things like that. At that time, there were a lot of qualifications you could do in the NHS, where you would be paid to train almost to get a postgraduate diploma and master's whilst working in the NHS. So I thought that might be another option. Then eventually, I got on at the University of Chester and did the postgraduate diploma to be a dietitian.

It was around the same time I'd just been accepted onto the dietitian postgraduate that the EIS was starting to have nutritionist roles. The EIS had advertised some apprenticeships including a few as a nutritionist and Nigel Mitchell actually contacted me asking if I would be interested in applying. So this was three years of applying to be a dietitian, having just been accepted, then this crops up with the EIS. I thought what do I do here? This sounds like it's going to be my dream role, but then I've invested all this time to get onto the dietitian training and I had been working as a clinical assistant dietitian.

So I kind of took the point and said, No, I'm gonna go down the dietitian route and hopefully those doors will open up for me later down the line. So I worked for quite a long time, as a dietitian. Doing all kinds of different rotations in different medical and surgical areas. I still had the aspiration to work as a sports nutritionist and would help out friends or recreational athletes training for triathlons etc. But it felt like I'd maybe missed the boat and I was now firmly in the clinical world of nutrition. I worked for a few years in the hospital. I had a break when me and my wife went travelling and we worked in India for a little bit, doing some teaching with a charity that works in the slums in Mumbai, which was quite good. It was like a nutrition and education charity. So that was a good little gap. When I came back, I then specialised in diabetes especially type 1 diabetes. I really enjoyed working with people to help them balance their insulin and nutrition. Due to my degree and interest in sport science I helped develop specialist services and education for athletes with type 1 diabetes. However, there was still the nagging desire to work solely in sport with elite athletes as a sports nutritionist. Then it was actually a job that came up while I was working in the NHS that pinged up and really grabbed my attention. I thought that that would be my dream job. It was the nutritionist for British Cycling leading into the Rio Olympics, I think it was in 2015 or 2016. I can remember being sat in an antenatal clinic in between patients reading the job description thinking, *"That's the kind of role I really want to be doing!"*

I applied, knowing that I didn't have the essential criteria, but I had a lot of experience as a dietitian. Obviously, I didn't get the job or even a reply. But I thought, yeah, that's the kind of job I wanted to be doing. I was getting a bit disillusioned with working in the NHS as I had been working there for more than 10 years now. So I kind of thought, right, I really need to think about what I need to do to get these kinds of jobs, that's where I really want to go.

I was thinking that I was probably going to have to do a master's and leave my career to make this leap to be a performance nutritionist. I was still seeing athletes on the side, you know, recreational people, and doing bits of volunteering. When I was doing my dietitian training, I did some voluntary work with Wrexham Football Club, who were in League Two at the time, and did a bit of volunteering with Warrington Wolves. So just going in and seeing people and hanging around and doing those bits of work there. Then I had a chance meeting with James Morton when I was presenting on the physiology and nutritional aspects of type 1 diabetes at conference. James Morton was there presenting about cycling physiology and his journey with Team Sky. I was aware of James obviously with the work he was doing with Team Sky and we got chatting and I was telling him where I was up to with my career. You know, I'm at this this crossroads, I really want to be working with top athletes like you are, kind of thing, but I'm stuck in the NHS, I've got a good job, I'm in my 30s and can't really see what I need to do next. James encouraged me to think about coming to Liverpool John Moores and doing the MSc in sports nutrition.

So I went up and had a meeting with James and Graeme Close and they told me about the master's and the opportunities that would probably crop up as a result of it so that's what I decided to do. So I lived off my wife's salary for a year and ditched my job in the NHS and did the master's. I struggled for a year; I took out a loan. Like I say, I lived off my wife's salary. So I went all in and then it's kind of worked out from there.

The plan was if I had to go back to the NHS, I could always go back with my tail between my legs but the plan was to get this master's and use it as a springboard then to work in professional sport as a nutritionist, ideally within endurance sport, road cycling and things like that. So that's kind of how I got there. I managed to get a placement during my master's with the EIS and British Cycling. So that was a big thing that allowed me to get my foot in the door and meet people and a job came up as a maternity cover nutritionist with British Para Swimming while I was still doing my master's. I didn't know anything about swimming or parasport but I thought it's a good opportunity and it really was.

So I applied and managed to get the job while I was still on the master's and then once I had a firm foot in the door then there were lots of other jobs and bit-part roles and small projects that cropped up in the EIS and I was always saying yes to everything. For example, I did some work with equestrian; I didn't have a clue about the sport or the horse world or any of that, but again, I learned a heck of a lot from a different culture, working with people that hadn't been exposed to nutrition or sports science before. I was still doing some voluntary work with a local boxing gym and some paid work with recreational and semi-pro athletes to supplement my part-time income with the EIS. The contacts and work that I did around the EIS and Olympic system led to me being recommended for more work here and there which kind of snowballed. I think it helped being a bit older and being a registered dietitian; it meant that people were more confident to pass referrals on to me and to put my name forward, and that I was able to take on the work.

And then bit by bit I have managed to take on more major and permanent roles in sport including senior nutritionist at British Cycling (EIS) and then nutritionist with Ineos Grenadiers cycling team which I did for two seasons. So I ended up following on from James Morton in the role he was doing when it was Team Sky. So it's like I managed to fulfil the two jobs that made me really decide to go "all in" for a career in sports nutrition. My two dream jobs, nutritionist with British Cycling and nutritionist with Team Sky. I've managed to do that quite quickly; that has all happened within the five years after getting my master's and now I'm head of nutrition for a team called Uno-X Pro Cycling Team.

After working with Ineos and providing consultancy to Uno-X for two years, I had to decide at the end of 2021 which team I was going to join full time. Uno-X are a Pro Tour team which is the level below World Tour where Ineos race. At first it wasn't an issue but as Uno-X have grown it started to become a conflict. So for the 2022 season, I moved to Uno-X full time as head of nutrition. I made the decision as it was much more appealing to help build and develop a system from scratch with complete autonomy and try and help Uno-X progress to the next level. I learned a lot in two seasons with Ineos but I was aware that, take away the status of the team, I wasn't going to get the same personal development and job satisfaction which I have now. So that's basically a whistlestop tour of my career to date!

**That's class. It's a journey that I wasn't aware of, which has been quite insightful there. So just to make sure I understood that and it kind of feeds into the second question, when you first got involved in nutrition, that was with the EIS placement opportunity underneath Nigel, would you say that was kind of your first nutrition exposure working with athletes?**

**James:** Yeah that would have been around the time I was aware of that so that would have been in 2007. Around the time, I was doing a little bit of volunteering with Wrexham Football Club and at Warrington Wolves rugby league (academy) as well. But again, I didn't have any reason to be there other than I was just starting my training to be a dietitian and I wanted to eventually work in sport. I was proactive and maybe a bit pushy; I knew the world of sport wasn't going to come and knock on my door so I thought that I would try and utilise any contacts I had to see what it was like and try and get my hands dirty. It's one of those things when you look back and actually think how unqualified I was at that time to think I should be working with professional athletes. But when you're young and ambitious, you think, well, I need to just get some experience. So I'll just go and see what the craic is and just nosy around and any contacts I can get and leverage, it will help. But the EIS internships or apprenticeships were kicking off around that time and that's when it looked like there actually could be a career path in being a performance nutritionist. It was a sliding doors moment as I had just been accepted to do the postgraduate dietitian diploma at the same time the EIS apprenticeships came out. I'm glad I went the way I did, but at the time it was hard to know what was the right way to go!

**Who are some of your mentors in your life and why?**

**James:** I have a few, within the team that I work in: our head of performance, a guy called Espen Aareskjold who's not a nutritionist, and he's come into the sport from quite an unconventional background. He worked as a mental health nurse and he's a coach on our team; he coaches riders, but he has a real good questioning mindset. He is very good at seeing problems from multiple angles and different scenarios. He's really good at provoking and challenging dogma. So he's somebody that I would say is a mentor to me. Nigel Mitchell has been a mentor to me a lot over the years as he has put me forward for lots of opportunities that I probably wouldn't have backed myself for. When I was first starting out working in cycling, he had a lot of experience with how it all worked on the ground and shared some of his learnings. I'd say probably early on in my journey James Morton was a mentor. He helped me through my master's and I think he appreciated the leap I was taking as we are a similar age, but also the skill set and personality that I had. I then worked under him with my role with Ineos and Science in Sport. He was a good mentor to have, and he helped me during my first Tour de France as he had experienced a lot of the same challenges in the same team a few seasons earlier. So yes, in my professional life, I would have to say that those three have been the main mentors that have guided me at various points.

**In terms of standout moments in your career so far, when I say that what's the top thing that comes to your mind?**

**James:** Yeah, I think for me, it would be doing the Tour de France in 2020. The Tour de France is like the pinnacle of professional road cycling. It's the pinnacle of things that I wanted to work in. I wasn't a cyclist growing up; I'm from a rugby league and football background. For me cycling was just what you did your paper round on, it wasn't a sport as such for me growing up, but I've kind of fallen in love with the sport, because of how important nutrition is. But doing that tour in 2020, after COVID, it was when COVID was still raging, the team I was working with at the time were in a bit of a transitional phase. There was so much scrutiny because of COVID, because of how the team were performing and the nutrition team that had just started that season. We were brand new and I was tasked with being the guy that went to the Tour de France. It probably shaped me; I learned a lot about myself, a lot about pressure, a lot about how I operate in different situations. It was really hard, probably the hardest professional thing I've ever done, but it's definitely a standout moment. I definitely came through that Tour de France as a better, more reflective practitioner. That would probably be the standout moment.

**How difficult was it with COVID, logistics, all of the scrutiny around how food had to be so tight during COVID? Was it just a mental time from a logistical point of view to actually be a nutritionist with all of those restrictions?**

**James:** Yeah, but then I was in the Tour de France. You've worked in football and rugby. It's the same as being in a rugby, or football World Cup final. But some of the guys on the team had never met in person. So I was then with these guys for almost a month where you're on the road with them, trying to optimise their nutrition and trying to understand them. Riders from different cultures. That was the riders and then there were other staff members that I was having to work with day in day out, room with, that I had not really had a chance to build any real rapport or connection with and that was tough.

The team during that season was in a bit of a transition; they'd won the Tour de France a lot the past 10 years and they'd won in the past two years. But then riders were on uncertain form and there were injuries and illness. We started as one of the favourites but quickly were on the back foot so everything was under massive scrutiny, including every practitioner. It was the same as if Barcelona or Manchester United suddenly started underperforming: everybody's kind of in the spotlight. In football it's the players and manager that get the scrutiny. In cycling, everything peripheral gets questioned: is it the equipment? Are the riders overtrained/undertrained, have they got their nutrition wrong and underfuelled? Are they too heavy or too light, etc etc.

That was intense, as well as having COVID because at that time, there were two tests and the team was expelled from the tour. So if you had two positive tests in the staff or rider group, the team was expelled. So you had one on the first rest day and then it was like this big sword of Damocles hanging over everybody. So everyone was scrutinising everything from that perspective. Rider performances hadn't gone to plan so everything's then under the microscope, which at that team it is anyway, but this felt like it was a few levels up. Luckily, I had James Morton, who I was speaking with daily and checked in with each day. But yeah, it was tough. Usually when things are tough, my response is to just try and work harder, try and do more, try and work harder. But it was one of those times that no matter how hard I worked, it wasn't getting any easier.

**What's the influential factor why you've been successful in your career? What is it that you've done to get where you are? So in that five-year journey from finishing your master's to working for one of the most successful cycling teams in the world and a governing body at the same time, what is it that you have got?**

**James:** Yeah, I was thinking about this not too long ago, because I'd had a 10-year journey before getting that first role. I felt that with the junior roles I was able to fast forward through. I had a lot of the softer skills. Then I was just building up my exposure to being in elite sport. The thing that I would say sets me apart was the fact that although there were a lot more clever academic people than me on my master's, I knew that if it was me and one other person and there was an opportunity, or there was me or anybody on my master's presented with an athlete or a coach in a high pressure situation, I would have the interpersonal skills to navigate that. I've had so many consultation hours over the years; I used to do an antenatal clinic with pregnant mothers from inner city Manchester and you'd have alcoholic mums turning up to antenatal clinics with diabetes, and you're in with the doctor and the midwife trying to advise them on their insulin and what they should be eating, and they've got substance issues; and working on a ward with you adjusting somebody's nutrition when they're being fed by a tube in the stomach, and they're unconscious, and the families are asking you why you're doing what you're doing and the consultant asking you the same! Just the ability to communicate with lots of complex people in mad situations and be able to adapt my style for the desired outcome is probably something that has maybe allowed me to adapt quite well to different situations in elite sport.

People at the top of sport, whether that be coaches or athletes, they're the outliers of their world; they are physiological freaks; they also are something different psychologically which makes them so successful and hungry. Being able to apply a lot of what I've learned from working as a clinical dietitian to that space is probably something that's helped me navigate quite well, building relationships, how to change my style to work with different individuals. Yeah, I'd say that's probably my strong point.

**And just a quick one to dive into working with one to ones there, which is such an important area of building that trust with athletes or individuals. What I see with some of the junior practitioners coming through is just that experience of knowing how to engage with the individual, meet them at their level, build that rapport quickly, the junior practitioners just don't have that yet. I think that comes from experience and it comes with practice, but in your mind, what are the key things to remember to nail that initial one to one with an athlete that you've never met?**

**James:** Yeah, I think you have to really try and assess where the athlete is at, not where the athlete is at with their nutrition knowledge or what you need to work on with the athlete's nutrition, but where they're at mentally so try and get to really understand them as a person. My approach with athletes is very collaborative. So it's very much what do we need to work on together? How can I help you? We've signed a really experienced rider this year and he's only a few years younger than me; he's won pretty much everything in professional cycling.

My first meeting with him, I asked what can I help you with? What do you want from me? And then that opens up an opportunity to get to know him a little bit, get to know he's got kids and his family setup and what he's actually interested in and use that as a bit of a way of going in. Whereas if I treated him like an 18-year-old, who had just joined our team, it may have been received wrong by the athlete. But you're really trying to understand that person before you then try and think, oh, I just need to dump everything I know about nutrition in this person's head and then that's my job done. Sometimes it might be a few consultations before you're actually working on detailed nutrition and trying to get them to change behaviour or action things.

I think that that's something that can often be missed, because you think, right, I've got limited time with this athlete, I just need to get across all my wisdom, all my biochemistry knowledge, blind them with science and then give them an infographic and then that's job done. That just doesn't work. In my experience, it's about understanding the person. I remember reading a paper a few years ago written about sport psychologists and how successful they are in having an impact (or not). A quote that stood out and resonated with me was, "They need to know you care, before they care what you know."

**I agree 100%. What has been one of your biggest challenges in your career so far? Maybe outside of that COVID situation?**

**James:** In terms of the biggest challenges, we spoke earlier about finishing a master's and I made it sound quite quick, but it's maybe only in the past year like this season and last season, it's probably the first time I've had just one job or one role. When I was with INEOS, I was still needing to do other work at the time. When I first did my master's and finished, it was two days here, one day there, voluntary work, so you are sacrificing a lot of family time.

We have weekends and evenings as time to build this kind of caseload and reputation and experience, so that eventually, you can then have a big substantive role, instead of needing to have five one-day-a-week roles that end up being more than that.

Early on, that was hard, managing my time, because there are a lot of nutritionists who are very good at being quite savvy, business wise, very good at dedicating the right amount of time to a project or a client, whereas I struggle to do that.

So I would have like 10 projects going on and I feel like I need to give all 10 projects 100% at all times, and then, eventually, something has to give and that's usually me who would then feel like I'm burning out because it's impossible to deliver that much to that many people. So learning how to manage my time and prioritise has been something that's been a challenge, especially in those early years, when you've got like 10 bosses, for example. I did feel like I couldn't say no to anything, because I was still new in the game and probably a bit insecure that the work would dry up. That was a big challenge early on. Learning to be a bit more selective with when it's okay to actually set boundaries and say no to things is important too.

**Yeah, that's probably me right now in my career, just taking too much on. What characteristics do you think people need to work in our industry of nutrition?**

**James:** In terms of personal characteristics, you need to be honest and deliver. Elite athletes get used to so many people coming in and out of their lives and they are busy, goal-oriented people, they have families, they have to train. So they quickly can figure out the people who are in it for their own gain and the people that are there to help them improve. Being honest and delivering on things that you say you're going to do is something that will make you successful.

Saying yes to everything and being open-minded to opportunities. It can be easy to focus on the negatives of a situation but being able to take a step back and think that this could actually be an opportunity. Like I said,

I've done voluntary work, that at the time, I obviously needed the money like we all do, but then that voluntary work has quickly opened up other doors, other connections, plus the learnings I took away from helping these athletes that had never had nutrition support before. Working with equestrian, for example. If somebody said, name your top 10 sports you want to work in, I didn't even know equestrian was a sport. But again, it then opened up other doors, other experiences, learning other cultures and the demands and challenges of different sports, things like that.

Being thorough and detailed. I was working with somebody recently and they accused me of being too detailed, and too thorough. It was somebody who's working alongside me and I'm actually line manager for them. I kind of said, well, if you want to work with me and in this, then this is how I work so if it is too detailed, then that's something you need to work on. Because that's how I work. Details matter, especially when you are working with elite athletes. Perhaps I am too detailed and too thorough, but I believe that that's probably what sets me apart that when I do something for a rider or for a project or for an athlete, it's done. Obviously I adjust the amount of detail that goes into the output that an athlete or coach sees as the end point. But the detail in analysis, planning, pre-mortem and evaluation is there. No stone is left unturned, and I know that, okay, I've done as much as I can on that.

**What would be the biggest recommendation to a new student entering the industry now? If you were to rewind, with all of the knowledge and experience you've got, if that was James doing a sports science degree or doing the master's, what would you be saying to yourself at that age?**

**James:** So it's something that I am still working on myself, but if you want to work in nutrition, you need to have a good understanding of how people engage with food. I know that sounds basic, but the way we're taught and the way we've been trained, it's all very science based and theoretical pathways, working with grams per kilo and things like that. But you need to have an understanding how people will engage with food when they go to a restaurant, how people engage when they go shopping, people's understanding around food and food culture. I've done a lot of jobs working in kitchens as a pot washer, bartender, waiter, working with hospital catering and kitchens as well.

But I wish I'd probably appreciated how much I learned from those experiences and maybe took more notes. When you are washing the pots in your local pub and seeing how people engage with food, and what food means to people and routines and rituals, that's something that I wish I'd taken more notice of. I learned to cook at a young age; I'd say now my cooking is still functional, but I wish I'd learnt some more fancy chef skills at a younger age.

The other thing I would say is any opportunity you get that's working with people is an opportunity that's going to make you a better sports nutritionist because it's all people management. What we do is get athletes to optimise or change their behaviour around food to improve performance. So, any experience around people is going to enrich that, whether that's on a night out, in the pub with your mates, whether that's working on a building site or doing different jobs, it's all working with different people from different walks of life and athletes or people from different walks of life too. You go into your changing room at Bristol, there'll be well-educated people who have probably gone to private school and then there's probably guys who've come up from a different background. So having exposure to different people is going to make you more successful at the pointy end of being a nutritionist.

Sometimes students will only want to do roles that are working in nutrition with athletes, and that can be quite narrow; you might be able to do something in nutrition with disadvantaged families, for example. I would say you'd probably gain a lot more experience and knowledge from that than you would delivering a PowerPoint presentation to some under-16 footballers who are not going to engage with it. Just not looking a gift horse in the mouth and trying to see every experience as an opportunity is something that's free CPD, if you like. That's one of the things when people ask me about work experience, or shadowing, I would always say, if you go into any boxing club in the country, any boxing gym and say, I'm studying nutrition, can I get involved, they would bite your hand off. Probably any amateur or domestic cycling club would have the same response.

I know you've worked with a lot of boxers and I've worked with one or two. But the stuff I learned with those guys who were professional boxers making weight, what they were currently doing, how I could help improve them, that's still stuff that I use now and reflect on. I know when I was doing it at the time, I was doing it for free. But it was free training for me, whereas I went into it thinking I've got carte blanche to do whatever I want with these guys to help as long as they make weight for this day and they feel good. So yeah, I learned a lot from that. So I always recommend people do that and the same with cycling, all of the cycling teams in the UK below the top level, they won't have any nutrition provision. So again, if you went in saying I'm studying a master's in sports nutrition, can I work with some of your riders? The answer is going to be yes. Then you learn by doing, you build relationships and that's kind of how it works. Too often people can be precious and think I'm just going to wait for this dream job at Man United or Team Sky and that just doesn't happen without building these connections and skills first.

**It's so funny that you mentioned that boxing club because when I moved to Bicester, there's an amateur boxing club here and I just wanted to help some more boxers out. So I put my head in and said to the owner of the club, who owns it, who runs it and he said it's me, why, what is it you want? I said exactly what you've said and I wasn't really looking for paid work if I'm honest, it was just that I wanted to support some local boxers in my town. I quite often tell that story to the people on my mentorship programme that the only reason he knew that I existed on this planet was because I went into the front door of the boxing club. Without that they just don't know you're there. But if you do it, you make the effort, nine times out of ten, as you know, they're going to accept some free work.**

**James:** And then, you know, when that dream job does come up, it's like, well, what experience have you got? And you can say I've been working with this professional boxer and we've done this. It's all stuff that you've done off your own back but it's so rich, because that's one of the reasons why I like working in cycling, weight making or sports where weight is important. It's so challenging as a nutritionist; it's a real fine line, because if you get it wrong, it can be your fault. But if you get it right, and you've worked with an athlete to nail the weight for a set date and they perform, then it's like a high risk, high reward. That's one of the reasons why I love working in cycling. I would work with more boxers in the future; when my current role maybe calms down a little bit, it's something I'd like to return back to because I like that feeling that you can plan and you've done everything and you think it's right, but it's still a little bit uncertain, you know, you're working with tiny margins, aren't you? So it's high risk but it's also really rewarding, knowing that you've done everything to make it right. Whereas in sports where nutrition isn't a key determinant of performance and body composition or weight making aren't as key components, it doesn't have that same buzz for me personally.

**There's definitely that buzz when the weigh-in day is coming. Are there any areas of nutrition that are not currently taught which you think are fundamental to learn? You touched on it earlier around that ability to get to know people quickly and stuff like that. But I know there's loads of behaviour change stuff. We're beginning to see a lot more courses in that now, but in the role that you're in, if you could go back and add a module into some of these degree programmes, what would that be?**

**James:** It'd be consultation skills and clinical reasoning. In my dietitian training, it wasn't all perfect dietitian training, but the thing that I thought was really good was just the hours and hours of consultations you did, both observing people and then doing them yourself or doing parts of consultation. So now for three or four clinics, you might just be introducing yourself, introducing the dietitian, going through the referral, setting up the scene and then handing over to the dietitian. So you're getting used to actually opening a consultation and then the next week, you might do that, and then you might be tasked with taking a history. Then you get some real brutal feedback from that. So the hours and hours of consultation skills that you get, as a dietitian, are invaluable. That was the big thing when I did my MSc in sports nutrition that I felt was missing. The knowledge I gained from all of the physiology, the biochemistry and the lab skills, all that kind of stuff was golden. But the consultation work and practitioner skills side are often missing on a lot of the MSc sports nutrition programmes. Those hours and the continual process of being appraised and somebody giving you feedback, and then reflecting on every consultation that we had to submit every week, was really valuable.

It was like five reflections that you had to go through with the supervisor at the end of each week and some of it was brutal. Some of it, you're sat there squirming in this consultation and the patient's being really awkward with you because you've come at it wrong, because you're not experienced and this patient's been given a diagnosis that they're upset about, and you've gone in too heavy footed thinking, "I just need to tell them what they need to eat."

Then you need to be rescued by the supervising dietitian, then they're having to step in and it's quite embarrassing, and at the time, you just want the ground to swallow you up. But with each one of those experiences, you learn so much from it. It's something that I feel quite strongly about, the professional standards and practitioner skills in how sports nutritionists are trained. I've been speaking with SENR and BDA about it and it's an area that I would like to be more involved with, supporting some of that professional practice side of things.

**Mate, that's gold. Nutrition is obviously progressing quite quickly. So in the next five years, obviously, we've now got the influence of AI, we've got technology, where do you think the discipline of nutrition will be in five years' time?**

**James:** What a question! I definitely think with technology and AI (I don't know enough about AI) it's only going to get bigger and as a profession we have to engage with it. I am always open to new developments and trialling them. Anything that can help with time management, organisation and take away some of the menial "data entry" tasks that nutritionists have to do is of interest. At the moment, there's loads of apps that can give you dietary recommendations and some of them are quite well tailored for sport. The big thing I don't like about a lot of them is that they're "black box". A lot of apps are algorithm based and developed with a lot of assumptions. Elite athletes don't fit into these standardised approaches. That has been where I've struggled, not having the ability to "override" and use your own judgement to adjust inputs and outputs.

Sometimes when you're working with these outliers, like professional cyclists who will do like 25-30 hours a week of training, the amount of carbohydrate they would eat in a training week or a racing week in my experience can "break" these algorithms. Then athletes are saying, it told me to eat this amount of carbohydrate, which is probably right. But then the protein and fat that I'm being told to eat is just way off and that's the key point. So having more nutritionists involved in the development of apps and technologies, so it can be really road tested because so much of it is designed for the average people training for a marathon or recreationally active. Nutrition is important but when you start putting in the numbers of the guys that we're working with, then that's where I think the problems lie.

So I think technology and apps and things like that are great. But it's that side of things that I'm always wary of. When we do a lot of trialling and testing new apps, softwares and technologies, after a bit of road testing, it always comes back to it's just not fit for purpose for our world at the moment. It can be quite dangerous with all of the sensors and wearables and things like that. It's something I have a big concern about in terms of now it's like you can measure everything and people just get blinded by data and numbers. You can measure everything but what does that mean? What can you infer with this data you've measured? Can you actually do anything with it? Is it just normal physiology? Should we even be bothered about the anxiety that it's causing? The additional stress of a "good" or "bad" value or response? Or should we just actually focus on the things we can control and we have a better understanding of? It's exciting and I'm always very curious but sceptical at the same time. You have to be because the day you just "pooh-pooh" anything new that comes along, that's when you'll get left behind. But if you're one of those people, if you're an early adopter, you have to be really rigorous with how you appraise these technologies and sensors before you put them in the faces of athletes because you'll quickly lose trust because the athletes will figure out that they're not fit for purpose quite quick.

**Have you had a play with Hexis? Have you road tested that with your guys and how did that fare?**

**James:** Yeah, early on so it's probably two years ago now, we did. Exactly that happened, we kind of said, look maybe for a strength and power athlete, maybe for a weekend warrior, but it's just not scalable for our guys at the moment. We gave them quite a lot of harsh feedback. I know Dr Sam Impey and Dr David Dunne quite well, so it was welcome feedback. It's something I'm going to pick up with them again soon just to see where it's up to now because that's one big thing for me, I have 30 riders so if you think 30 riders all needing 30 plans with the way it works in professional cycling, you might have three races going on at the same time in three different countries. So then the analysis and plans for those riders in those races is just a lot of work. So I'm always open to anything that could save some of that time and data entry and automate some of it. Yeah and just free up more time then for working on the actual behaviour change side of things and engaging with the athlete using the data as a starting point and then using my skills to then help the athlete use that data to make changes. I am currently working on an in-house app with our current team systems and data scientist, as so far other than my spreadsheet, I've not managed to find anything "off the shelf" that is better!

**Right, we've got the last three questions; they're normally a little bit quickfire. So is there a book that you would recommend? It doesn't really have to be nutrition based, have you read a book recently that you enjoyed, and you're happy to share?**

**James:** Yeah, I've started reading a bit more this last year. Since my little boy is now sleeping a bit better, you can probably resonate with this, I am reading a bit more before I go to bed instead of just passing out because I'm going to be woken up every few hours. Yeah, a book that I read quite recently, which was a gift, was called *Out Of Thin Air* by Michael Crawley. It's about elite Ethiopian marathon runners and a competitive runner and anthropologist from the UK that went and lived and trained with them. It's actually more of the social, cultural side of things, the philosophy of these guys and how they live their lives rather than the sports science and the fact that they were born and live at altitude. So that was a really good book just about how simply they lived their lives and their cultures and their beliefs and that human side of things. So that was a book I've read recently that was a really good read, so I'd recommend that one. Another one is a book that I really liked the title of. I've only read it a couple of times, *The Score Takes Care of Itself* by a guy called Bill Walsh (and others). That's something we speak about all the time with athletes; let's focus on the behaviours and the routines and the structures and then the outcome will mostly take care of itself. So that's more of a sport, philosophy management kind of book.

**What key principles do you follow every day that keep you operating at gear six?**

**James:** I try and exercise regularly; that sounds quite obvious but for me, it's as much mental as physical. Just getting out as often as you can to run or to be active. I think mentally that that's essential. For me personally, when I've had busy periods, where that's been the thing that I've maybe sacrificed a little bit, the quality of my work suffers. Probably my mental focus suffers and probably being a good husband and a good father suffers. So yeah, being active as often as possible.

Working as hard as you can, all of the time. It sounds obvious but just trying to work as hard as you can all the time. I've always felt that when I played sport, I wasn't the most gifted physically, I wasn't the fastest, most skilful or the strongest rugby league or football player, but I always knew I'd be selected because I would graft and I would work and get stuck in and challenge. I've adopted that in my work life, as well as in my professional life. Always deliver on the promises you make as well, so if you say you're going to do something, you have to do it.

**Final question, in your eyes and your experience, what makes a successful performance nutritionist in sport?**

**James:** I think to be a successful performance nutritionist in sport, you have to really love it. You have to really be thinking about it 24/7. It is a job but you need to be always looking out on the horizon. You always need to be thinking about what's the new thing that's coming. What's the athlete going to ask me next week? What have they read about on social media? You always have to be ahead of the curve. To do that you have to love it; it can't be a grind to be reading a new paper or reading a blog that some athletes put out about some hocus-pocus supplement.

You have to constantly be thinking about it. It's your passion as well as your job; you have to really be into it. It's not something you can dip your toe in, because performance sport is all-consuming for the athletes we work with; it's all-consuming to be a specialist working in that area; the way you approach nutrition should be the same in my opinion. The top athletes that you work with, they're optimising everything with the training, how they live their life, all those other things, so they expect their S&C coach is the best in their area, is the most up to date. He knows everything there is to know about lifts and techniques. They expect their nutritionist is the best nutritionist, you know; they should be ahead of the curve, they should know what things are and that's kind of how I approach it. I think that as a student, that's how you should be thinking as well. If I want to work with elite people then I need to think of how I can be the best sports nutritionist I can be. I've not really thought about that before I spoke about it but yeah, that's probably something I would say.

**That's golden, absolutely golden. That's the end of the interview, so thank you so much.**

## JAMES'S THOUGHTS

The persistence James showed in the pursuit of his dietitian's qualification at the University of Chester is a reminder to us all to keep trying! Additionally, he's another leading nutritionist who volunteered early on in his career whilst at Wrexham and Warrington Wolves, a club I know very well!

I admire James's braveness, living off his wife's salary and ditching the NHS to study the MSc at LJMU. This was a career-defining decision and one which has worked wonders. Another example of jump and the net will catch you!

I love how James refers to his interpersonal skills as a key aspect, he believes, of his success. Whether it is the alcoholic mother from Manchester or a leading world tour cyclist, our ability to connect with the human opposite us and have a meaningful conversation with them is part of a successful strategy.

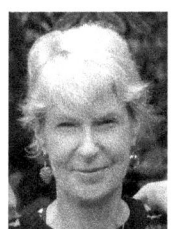

# CHAPTER 8:
# *PROFESSOR LOUISE BURKE*

Louise is a sports dietitian with 40 years of experience in the education and counselling of elite athletes. She worked at the Australian Institute of Sport for 30 years, first as head of sports nutrition and then as chief of nutrition strategy. She was the team dietitian for the Australian Olympic teams for the 1996–2012 Summer Olympic Games. Her publications include over 350 papers in peer-reviewed journals and book chapters, and the authorship or editorship of several textbooks on sports nutrition. She is an editor of the *International Journal of Sport Nutrition and Exercise Metabolism*. Louise was a founding member of the Executive of Sports Dietitians Australia and is a director of the International Olympic Committee Diploma in Sports Nutrition.

She was awarded a Medal of the Order of Australia in 2009 for her contribution to sports nutrition. Louise was appointed as Chair in Sports Nutrition in the Mary MacKillop Institute of Health Research at Australian Catholic University in Melbourne in 2014 and took up this position in a full-time capacity in 2020.

It was an absolute honour to interview Louise for this book. Her wisdom, views and overall openness to share experience for this book are superb. I know you will enjoy reading this chapter as much as I enjoyed doing the interview.

You can follow Louise on:
Twitter @LouiseMBurke

---

**The first question that I ask everyone is who are you and what are you up to right now in the world of sports nutrition and applied physiology?**

**Louise:** I'm Louise Burke, chair of sports nutrition at Mary MacKillop Institute for Health Research at Australian Catholic University (ACU). I've moved into academia as a full-time researcher, as possibly the last page of my career in sports nutrition. This comes after a background of 40 years as a practitioner involved with elite athletes in various phases and opportunities. Most of this work was undertaken at the Australian Institute of Sports (AIS) where I undertook research as a "hobby", to find evidence to underpin the practices of our sports nutrition team. Looking back, however, these research activities often provided a special interaction with athletes, and the sharing of resources that we wouldn't have otherwise had. I've only just come to recognise that the activity or process of doing research is sometimes as important as the outcomes of the project.

**And with the dietetics and the nutrition, how and when did you first get involved in that area of research?**

**Louise:** It was a complete accident! I had absolutely no idea when I was finishing school of what I wanted to be. I enjoyed studying science and was accepted to study medicine at university, but at the last moment I changed my mind and reverted back to a simple science degree. I couldn't see myself being a doctor and I didn't want to take a place from somebody who really did. I thought if I started with a science degree, I could change it later into something that sparked my interest. I didn't know that it was possible to study nutrition, but gravitated to some subjects in food technology that were offered by the university. Although these subjects weren't "quite right", I realised that I was interested in food, which made me notice the publicity for the creation of a new university in my state – Deakin

University – which offered a dietetics course. So I changed universities in the middle of the year to study nutrition, still not realising that there was a career path as a dietitian. Luckily, I was offered a position at the end of the degree to undertake their graduate diploma of dietetics and it seemed a great option to apply my nutrition knowledge.

The spark for converting this into a focus on athletes and sports nutrition, again, was another "lucky break". Our course was small – 20 students – and we were invited to the home of the course convener, Dr Richard Read, for a meal. There, I noticed that he was only eating lettuce and cheese and I questioned him about his food choices. He told me that he was running a marathon at the end of the week, and was applying some new research from Scandinavian researchers to his preparation. He explained that their study showed that if you depleted muscle glycogen with a low carbohydrate diet for a couple of days, then switched to a high carb intake at the end of the week, you could super-saturate your muscle glycogen stores, prolonging your optimal running pace for a longer period. That information exploded in my brain and joined up my mad passion for sport with my new skills in nutrition. There was no pathway to study this formally, but I had found "my person". I nagged Richard into letting me drop microbiology, and do a unit of "research" with him where we essentially read scientific papers and discussed ideas for translating this into sports nutrition practice. That was really the start of the whole thing.

**Great story. What was your first exposure to the elite sporting environment from a nutritional point of view?**

**Louise:** The dietetic course was a very crammed unit of study with placements over a 12-month period in order to meet the requirements of dietetic registration. But it required us to move to Melbourne where most of the hospitals were located. While I was doing this, I wrote to the Australian Rules football club that I follow (St Kilda). Australian Rules is a very old professional sport and the biggest team sport in Australia. My team is known for being hopeless – in the 150 years of its existence in the league, it has won the premiership (championship) exactly once. Actually I wrote to the best player in the club – Trevor Barker – who had the status of David Beckham in Australian Rules. I told him that nutrition was the missing link in allowing the Saints to win another championship and that I was the person who could bring this piece to the club. Later, when I was working at the club, I would see the fan mail that he received each week, mostly from young girls and not related to nutrition. But Trevor actually read my letter and passed it on to the club doctor, who rang me and invited me to contribute my expertise to the club. And that was the start of my career.

I look back now and see that I was ill-prepared for the task and for the 1980s culture of team sport. But it started the passion for wanting to bring nutrition to the attention of athletes. Knowing that there wasn't a career pathway or professional recognition for such work meant that I had to make my own. Those early years were about me nagging people in sports medicine centres and sporting clubs to be given an opportunity, and relying on the generosity of others. Then eventually, an opportunity at the AIS presented itself. Their original iteration of sports science/medicine included nutrition as an offshoot of the department of physiology. However, in the second phase of expansion, they realised that nutrition was its own speciality and needed dedicated expertise. I was lucky to be offered the role, and AIS sports nutrition developed from there for 28 wonderful years.

In reflecting on this, I can see that I've had a completely random career pathway. However, when time has passed and you get to look at it in reverse, it all makes sense. When you're living in the moment, things can feel frustrating and you often feel impatient that it's not happening quickly enough. But you just have to trust that everything you do contributes to your journey. Nothing is a waste of time because it is all going to teach you something and move you towards the destination from which you can look back with insight.

**Yeah, yeah. Very pertinent for me at the moment, where I am with my life and some of the decisions I'm having to make. Are you still in touch with Trevor now?**

**Louise:** No, Trevor died at 49 years old from cancer and I didn't ever have a chance to thank him for his role in my career. But in 2006, I had the opportunity to consult to the Saints, again (no, they still haven't won another premiership). When I went back to the club, it was exactly the same as I'd left it, an under-resourced stadium and ancient clubrooms. But Trevor's father Jack – now in his 80s – had been to every training session and game over that whole period. So, I had lots of opportunities to just hang out with him and chat about Trevor. I used to organise hot soup after some training sessions, and I would get him to serve it to the players because he was adored at the club. He was an old-fashioned gentleman and I don't think he understood science or appreciated how Trevor had changed my life. But he would tell me over and over about Trevor coming home from the club to the family dinner, saying how important it was to eat vegetables. It was really nice to be able to complete that circle.

**So for yourself, who were or are some of your biggest mentors in your life? And why have they been important for you?**

**Louise:** That's a great question. When I started there wasn't a career path that would allow me to contact people and say "How did you get there? What did you learn that made you able to work in this space?" I didn't have that opportunity. I think my mum and dad have been incredible mentors to me in ways they don't appreciate. Neither went to university, so they didn't have experience to help with my studies or even know what to study. But I grew up in a family of five children who appeared within a seven-year timespan, so that was a pretty busy household. From my parents and siblings, I learned to be organised and the importance of being generous, collaborative, and optimistic. So they gave me a lot of tools to work with, and attitudes and values to life that have been really important.

Studying dietetics at Deakin University in the 1980s didn't involve any formal education around exercise. So I basically had to fill in those gaps about exercise biochemistry and physiology through personal learning. I've received incredible generosity and support from people like Ron Maughan, and Mark Hargreaves, really robust exercise scientists who opened up the area to me and gave me opportunities well beyond what I deserved. And of course, the AIS was a wonderful environment, full of really special people who radiated passion and commitment. Every coach and athlete I've ever worked with has been a mentor; you learn so many things about the art of performance, as well as the science of performance from these people. The AIS was a hothouse of incredible sports scientists with whom I got to rub shoulders and learn from. There's too many to name, but Dave Martin is one who personifies the best of sports science to me. He continues to be really important in my life, because my love of working with him means that we will find ways to do this wherever our careers and lives take us. He's so positive and innovative, and has great showmanship. But behind the pizzazz, he has a really deeply founded understanding of science and sports science, as well as a great curiosity about what makes people tick. He makes it fun to do great work and learn new things. Then, there's my husband, John! How lucky is it to have a husband with so much expertise in exercise and nutrition! Even though he's now mostly applying it to community health and disease interventions rather than my frivolous areas of sports performance, I get constant support and information there. And finally, I have to acknowledge the biggest mentors of my life – all the young sports dietitians and sports scientists that are past members of AIS sports nutrition or my new little team at ACU. Too many to name and I wouldn't want to miss any of them – I don't think I have ever had a "dud" within the group. I'm being outshone by so many of them and love looking at the ways they're achieving their own sports nutrition careers. I can just sit back and be pulled along by the momentum of what they do. They have all made me a better person and practitioner.

**In your career, what would you say has been a standout moment or moments? And that can be applied? It can be research?**

**Louise:** There's "standout" moments in terms of good and bad. Good standouts aren't so much a single occasion, but a rolling existence of doing things that always keep you excited and challenged. This week, we've just finished a five-week research-embedded training camp as a collaboration between Australian Catholic University, the AIS Female Performance and Health Initiative and the National Rugby League Women's programme. We worked with First Nations female rugby league players, so I had the incredible opportunity to expand my cultural awareness of our Aboriginal and Torres Strait Islander people. But watching my incredible postdoc, Alannah McKay, pull over the most challenging of studies was incredibly rewarding. I was there to contribute a few skills in the actual delivery of the project, but just watching her take on the leadership role was fantastic.

Another one of my PhD students, an old AIS team member, Bronwen Lundy, received the news yesterday that her PhD has been passed with minor amendments, and her main paper has been chosen by *Medicine & Science in Sports & Exercise* to be a feature for their next edition. That's fantastic success because Bron works full time as a sports dietitian embedded with Rowing Australia and her work has been wholly applied in every sense of the word. She was able to integrate monitoring work and a clever intervention over the course of an Olympic cycle, providing value to the athletes she works with as well as being recognised scientifically. Every week there are little and bigger triumphs like this, where I get to enjoy my sports nutrition family making its mark.

But in terms of "bad standout", I think, the moment I realised that I needed to leave the AIS was a seminal experience, because it was an acceptance of failure for me. I finally got to the point of realising that I wasn't valued there; I wasn't effective. I recognised that I'd come up short, number one, but also that I should have realised it much earlier. I'd been deluding myself that you can change things if you just keep trying. But the reality is that you can't make people love you if they don't, and you can't make people value you when they don't. It was a giant wake-up call to recognise that just because I think I have lots to offer and receive positive feedback in other spheres, it doesn't mean it's a shared concept. It's confronting to finally realise that your dream environment doesn't feel the same way about you, but there's freedom in making the decision to move to somewhere or something where your value is reflected. I've been so lucky to have a new adventure provided to me by Australian Catholic University, where I can start again with a small team and reinvent myself.

I hope it's useful to share such experiences with young people. It's easy to look at people who amass lots of entries on their CVs and imagine that they're always riding the wave perfectly from success to success. I'm sure people would have thought, oh, the AIS has been so successful and Louise has been there forever, so they must adore her and everything she does. But it isn't always like that. Things can change, and your value and reputation can suddenly be meaningless in an environment. Recognising that I was a failure – by insisting on being in an environment that did not want me – was a standout moment, I think. My stupidity was not thinking about it like that earlier, and making an earlier decision to move on.

**Yeah, look, thanks for sharing that. You're the first person to provide a bad or a negative standout moment there. So that will be really valuable. My second question linked to that, was the moment that you had made that decision or accepted that, was it a relief for you?**

**Louise:** Oh, absolutely. It was an interesting situation, because I was completely aware that the AIS had changed. They had moved away from the direct preparation of athletes years earlier, and then after excruciating years of review, they dissolved sports nutrition and sports science. No more AIS sports nutrition after 28 years of (I thought) being world leaders in our field. I was invited to stay on in a new role as chief of nutrition strategy, which sounds important, but the reality was really frustrating. I had no agency, I had no resources. I asked lots of questions about the new goals of the AIS to see how I could contribute. I kept proposing various projects, but I would get knocked back all the time. I was successful in getting external grants to run ever more elaborate research-embedded training camps – e.g. our Supernova series – and thought that this was a novel way to keep working directly with athletes and coaches, while also advancing sports science/nutrition. But I didn't realise how poorly these were viewed within the AIS hierarchy. I kept persisting, thinking that if I worked harder and brought in more resources, that I would be respected. Even up to the conversation that made me realise the futility of this approach, I was still convinced that I had the power to do work that was appreciated. It took some harsh reflection from the AIS chief medical officer David Hughes to make me realise that the only thing that remained at the AIS was my dignity.

At one level, that was a huge gut punch and led to many tears. But the next morning, I woke up knowing that it was the best and most honest advice that I'd been given. I consider David to be a good friend, and I thank him for having the bravery to be straight with the information I needed to hear.

**Now, don't get too caught up on the definition of successful in this next question, but what do you think has been the most influential factor as to why you've had the career you've had in terms of your success?**

**Louise:** There is a lot of luck in life – being at the right place at the right time. Of course, you make a lot of luck yourself by working hard and seeking opportunities to be in the right place. I had the opportunity to think about what underpins success when the AIS came up with a set of four values that it wanted to promote within its workforce. You needed to be relentless, ingenious, exceptional and daring. We all had to pick a lanyard to state publicly which of these values you aspired to. I found it a bit confronting to choose one at first, because in Australia you don't want to be "up yourself" by running around telling people how good you are. I tried to settle on the one that was least "self-promoting", if you like. I went with "ingenious" because I thought you could be a bit self-deprecating in describing yourself like an evil mastermind in a Marvel film. But it got me reflecting on what it meant, and I found that I quite liked the aspiration of being ingenious. And that maybe my superpower is in creating ecosystems where people and resources gather to create magic.

Serendipity is one of my favourite words because I believe if you build an ecosystem with the right ingredients, incredible stuff can flourish because of all the interactions and energy. As I think back over the "successful" things I've done, a common element was putting wonderful people together with time and resources and permission to be great. That was certainly the secret to AIS sports nutrition and some of the projects we undertook. But more recently, our research-embedded training camps have thrown athletes, coaches and sports scientists into a little bubble away from the rest of the world, with opportunities to work together and learn or do new things. So many magic outcomes and stories have come from these little ecosystems – much more than the sum of the parts. I think what's contributed to my success, and my ability to keep being excited by my passion for sports nutrition, is that I've stumbled onto the secret of creating little ecosystems that are ignited by sparks – both planned and random. The success is very much a joint outcome – it's not my success. I've just contributed to providing a sort of lucky space full of incredible people and the spark to make it engage.

**I like what you're describing; the community of people working towards the same goal is a valuable point. In terms of challenges in your career, you have obviously shared some of the stuff there?**

**Louise:** Yeah, challenges for me come from the barriers that prevent you from fulfilling your potential and from scenarios of not being appreciated or understood. But sometimes, these challenges form part of the spark that ignites the ecosystem. Many of the best projects we have undertaken didn't occur because someone drove up and said, "Here's a million bucks and everything you need – go and do something." Rather, we plotted and scrounged and used ingenuity to find ways of getting loaves and fishes to turn into a meal. If you can be creative and think outside the envelope, and then find "your people" with similar values, success won't be far away.

Another challenge or frustration comes from being stuck in a structure where others have a different idea of what success looks like. I think success is achieved through teamwork and a supportive structure, but there's a cliched trope that sport is about relentless toughness. When I got to do my farewell speech at the AIS (it was during COVID so nobody was there listening to it), I suggested to the AIS that it needed to add a fifth value to its set. Kindness. I reflected on binge-watching *The Last Dance* (Netflix documentary) like everyone else did from their COVID lockdowns. It is clear that Michael Jordan was a great athlete, but the characteristics he portrayed in that show are not necessary, or the recipe, for success. I have seen many people who are the best in the world at what they do and have witnessed that they can achieve greatness without being a dick. Terrorising people to do better is not my idea of leadership. Collegiality and random acts of kindness achieve so much more than bullying.

**Characteristics of people who work in performance nutrition, or dietetics: if you were employing people in an organisation now, what are the key traits that you're looking for outside of kindness?**

**Louise:** The ability to be truly collaborative is important – a mindset to work hard on improving the group or the whole, as well as yourself. We talk about passion but it's a bit of a cliche in sport, because everybody describes themselves like that. I'm more interested in doing work that is underpinned by solid scientific knowledge and grounded in ethics. There's a certain need to be engaging and charismatic if you work in professional sport, where people like shiny things, but I want substance behind the showmanship. So I'm drawn to people who are clever, thoughtful and insightful, and on a continual journey of improving themselves. They want to learn more, take a deep dive into the science and evidence, and then translate it into innovative practice. It helps to have the ability to engage with people and to make your work feel fun and exciting, but the full package needs to have a sound underpinning.

**If you were entering the industry now, what would be the biggest recommendation? We've got a forever growing expansion of nutritionists and there are limited jobs, certainly here in the UK, in terms of sports clubs and in the big clubs it's becoming more and more difficult for some of these people to get jobs. So what would be your biggest recommendation to those entering the industry?**

**Louise:** Be collegial. I think there are two types of people in the world. There are those who think that success is a limited commodity; they feel envious and angry if somebody else is successful, because they think it diminishes their own opportunities. I'm part of the other group who thinks that success is an infinite commodity. There's plenty to go around and we can work together to share the opportunities.

Part of that thinking is to have a growth mindset that means that you're always willing to learn and become better, rather than being protective and insular about what you do. It's also about having a growth mindset for your colleagues – encouraging them also to become better rather than needing to outshine them and contain their achievements. Being creative to carve your own niche is important. There weren't jobs for me when I started my career, but I found ways to make myself valuable to others. I still believe that there are new opportunities out there in which people can create their own adventures.

It's a matter of continually exploring little opportunities – backing yourself to crack the code and having patience while you are doing it. As I said before, when you get somewhere and look back, it will all make sense. I've seen great case studies from some of my former team members from AIS sports nutrition who've carved new niches by spotting new opportunities and investing their creativity there. For example, Alicia Edge moved to a country area after leaving the AIS – outside the reach of professional sport.

So, she started an online platform for sports nutrition business, which does a lot of online counselling, but provides other services to athletes through electronic pathways. When COVID came along, she was able to pivot her investment into an expanded infrastructure that suited the new environment. Her business is now flourishing, thanks to canny insight into a different way to work under changed circumstances.

**I quite often tell some of the students now that when I moved to where I live with my wife, we didn't know anyone here. But I love the sport of boxing and so I went into the amateur boxing club and just spoke to the manager of the club and said, out of interest, have you got any fighters that would like to make the weight a little bit safer, and there were about six of them that put their hands up straightaway. But without going into that club, I would never have known this area.**

**Louise:** Yes, everybody thinks that they want to go to the Olympics. But whether you get there as an athlete, or as a sports nutrition practitioner, it takes years of hard work to hone your skills to that level. You have to start at the bottom, and collect knowledge, experiences, insights and confidence. The experience that you just described is a perfect example of finding a fingerhold and working your way up. At the start, you're getting just as much value from the interaction with the athletes you're working with, because the learning experience is just as real for you. As you accumulate your skills, the balance might change, but even at the top of your trade, each encounter with an athlete or sport is still a chance to learn.

**So going back to when you studied and what you know now, within your career, are there areas that you didn't learn as a student that have actually been incredibly valuable for you as a researcher or practitioner and as the lady that you are in the industry?**

**Louise:** I didn't have the chance to study exercise physiology or sports science in a systematic and organised fashion, so I've had to learn that myself in an ad hoc way. If I had my time again, doing a double degree which integrated nutrition and exercise from the start would have been really helpful. Sometimes, ad hoc learning is tough – especially when the penny suddenly drops on something and you realise that an earlier understanding would have made your work so much better. But on the other hand, the expectation that you need to improve your knowledge can sometimes allow you to gain more than you bargained for – and more than what might have been gained by learning in a linear path. I certainly feel "undercooked" in practical lab skills because there are lots of tests or equipment that I can't handle myself. When I set up studies, I'm reliant on other people to collect that data. So I value the opportunities to work with people who excel in the knowledge and practice of these tests, who can be trusted to be meticulous in their work.

**The industry of nutrition and dietetics, in five years' time, where do you think it will be? The reason I ask this is because the way that the world is developing at the moment at a very quick rate, how do you think that's going to impact nutrition?**

**Louise:** I think sports nutrition will develop with increasing technology and increasing specialisation. We already have access to gadgets and wearables that measure things and provide an overwhelming amount of information. The important breakthrough, however, will be in learning how to manage and interpret that information correctly so that it can be integrated into a holistic sports nutrition plan. This will mean cutting through the hype to identify what's really important and valuable, rather than what looks shiny and amazing.

But at the opposite end, I think sports nutrition will grow around really foundational areas of food and behaviour. ACU recently started a dietetic course from scratch. When I heard about it, I thought, ah, please don't make it another degree that specialises in sports nutrition; there are already tons of these. I'm not saying they're not good – in fact, they're great. But, as you said, they're producing a lot of people with a similar skill set who will have to think about where their next job is going to be in the traditional sports market. I was pleased to see that ACU went with a culinary nutrition focus – developing dietitians who have better skill sets in food service and food behaviour. It's ironic because when I studied dietetics, I considered the food service units and placements to be a side issue. I thought, I'm a scientist, I don't need to know this stuff. I am afraid I treated it with a lower level of attention and interest. This backfired of course; I've spent the rest of my career struggling with the logistics of feeding groups of athletes – whether in practice scenarios or in research camps – and in understanding how to construct menus and recipes to suit special diets or dietary interventions. I am also getting interested in understanding what drives dietary choices and compliance to dietary advice. It's exciting to see where clever technology can lead us. But at the end of the day, athletes eat food based on unique decision-making. How to understand and influence the grassroots of eating is the key to the practice.

**Yes, it's personal, and the best recruitment I've done, I think, in my whole career has been in the last six months where we've recruited a genuine sports chef who is unbelievably passionate about the food that he's delivering but he's got that personable character that he can connect with a rugby player in 10 seconds. We've completely transformed the club's view on what performance nutrition is. He's been instrumental in that and it's been amazing. There's a key marker that I, whether it's right or wrong, look at and it's how long do athletes spend at the dining table once they've finished their food. I always think about a really nice restaurant; you don't normally want to leave it that soon, because you're enjoying the environment, you've had a really nice meal, you're there with your friends, and you're taking in that social experience. I look at the players now when they finish their dinner; they're very happy, they're very content. They will sit there and they will talk and more often than not, it's "How good was lunch today? That was amazing." A few months ago it was about getting that in as quick as possible and off they go.**

**I just wanted to share that we've got the England women's rugby team currently in New Zealand for a World Cup. There was talk of me going over there and travelling, but obviously I had my commitments here. But the female nutritionist that we sent has actually got a chef background. So for me, she was this perfect combination of two disciplines where she was trained as a chef; she spent years in the kitchen. She knows all about food and now she's learned under Graeme and James. Like what better person to be placed over the other side of the world, where she can if she needs to dive in the kitchen and cook up some home comforts for the girls, she can do that straightaway.**

I say to my chef all the time now, is there a genuine chef course that nutritionists could do over here? And he always just says to me that the best way to learn is to just jump in the kitchen with me so I am trying to get in there as much as I can.

The last three are quickfire questions. Louise, is there a book that you've recently read, which improved your practice and it doesn't have to be nutrition, it could just be anything?

**Louise:** At the moment, I'm fascinated with evolutionary aspects of food and exercise and I've recently read books by Dan Lieberman (*Exercised*) and Herman Pontzer (*Burn*). They provide other perspectives on how we evolved to exercise and eat. I'm really interested in applying this insight to our current interest in low energy availability and REDs. At the moment, we see any situation of low energy availability as being problematic and causing a fixed set of problems. But, if you look at it from an evolutionary perspective, our ability to partition where we spend our energy in our bodies when there's a period of energy scarcity – and the flexibility with which we can do it in the context of age, sex and many other factors – is a hallmark of our success as a species.

I also love reading novels to keep me happy and across art and culture. My most recent favourite was *Lessons in Chemistry* (Bonnie Garmus), which features a female chemist who was unappreciated as a scientist until she got her own television cooking show. It was set in the 50s and 60s when a woman's place was in the home. But she achieved success by treating housewives as fellow scientists, and discussing meal preparation as a series of chemical reactions.

**Are there any key principles that you follow every day?**

**Louise:** My starting five: do some exercise, enjoy food, be kind to the people around you, have some fun and learn something new. Continual evolution is important, in the way you think and the way you practise.

**Nice. And to finish, in your view what makes a successful performance nutritionist?**

**Louise:** If I had to choose one thing, I still think it's teamwork. Humility, being confident in your work but not to the point that it overshadows other people.

## JAMES'S THOUGHTS

First things first, I love how Louise Burke getting involved in nutrition was a complete accident! Secondly, Louise provides a stunning example of being brave, going direct and reaching out to the best player of the club to inform him that nutrition is the missing link for the club to be successful.

I often discuss with mentees being brave and going direct when speaking to people. This is important when trying to get volunteer experience or work. Do not assume people know what you are after; tell them directly what it is you are messaging them about!

Huge respect to Louise with her standout moment. The first thing she mentioned was a training camp with Alannah McKay, a previous student and now colleague.

One of my favourite parts of this interview is when Louise speaks about serendipity. Her words here are true and struck a chord with me when I interviewed her.

I must finish on Louise's view of what makes a successful performance nutritionist... teamwork!

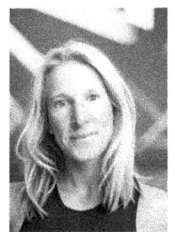

## CHAPTER 9:
## DR DANA LIS

Dana has over 15 years' experience working in performance nutrition and is heading into her fourth season with the Golden State Warriors NBA team (2018, 2022 NBA Champions). Her research in the department of Neurobiology, Physiology, and Behaviour (University California Davis, Baar Lab) has enabled the ideal integration of her research-based nutrition strategies.

Having studied her PhD at the University of Tasmania before her post-doctoral research position at University of California Davis, Dana has a brilliant background in both academics and the applied work. Whether it is elite cycling, soccer, global supplement companies, Olympic sports or basketball, Dana has the experience.

I have never met Dana in person but was fully aware of her work with Keith Baar following a visit to his laboratory a few years ago. I have read and cited her work in many applied case studies with players and it was a pleasure to dive into the journey of such a varied and exciting career.

You can follow Dana on Twitter @SummitFuel

**Dana:** Thanks for connecting and having me on this. It's awesome that you're sharing this type of invaluable professional insight. I'm excited to be part of it.

**All good. What is your background and for you, where did it all start?**

**Dana:** I think my background is probably a little atypical from a lot of people working in elite sport or in research and in sport. I am probably living proof that a person changes their career three times in their life. I started off completely opposite of anything science related. I didn't want to go to university. I was into art, music, climbing, outdoors stuff, and kind of a punk for a while. I did grow up figure skating but when that ended flipped the narrative, grew dreadlocks and started a rock climbing obsession. I was every mishmash of personalities you could imagine. With this my first career was in the outdoor industry. I was working towards becoming a certified rock-climbing guide and worked seasonally as an Outward Bound instructor in Colorado and in Costa Rica in global development projects. Being a group leader in those situations taught me so much of the emotional intelligence and people management skills that have been crucial to working in various sport environments.

The transient backpack lifestyle, while it was exciting for a few years, wasn't a long-term lifestyle for me. Some people can do it their whole lives and kudos to them. I am still envious when stories pop up of old friends still dirtbagging the world climbing. For me, I did not want to live out of a backpack and I found that after some years of maturing I needed an intellectual challenge. My partner at the time and now husband has always been and is still a hardcore academic.

I ended up going back to university at 22 years old. I went through college and then university. At that time in Canada you couldn't go to uni unless you did the base courses (grade 13) in high school. I chose not to do that in high school so had to take the 00 levels college courses to eventually apply and get accepted into the University of British Columbia. I ended up in sciences, then nutritional sciences and then part of the sought-after small cohort of dietetic specialisation.

So, I went from total punk to being able to get into a highly reputed programme. I didn't connect with a lot of people at uni because most students were just fresh out of mom and dad's house and I was at a much different point in my life. I had to work and also started racing bikes so I was locked into school and that was it. Having what you call in the UK "a gap year(s)" was what I needed to be mature and successful to know exactly what I wanted to do for the next career. Once in dietetics, I found sport nutrition and was yeah, was just completely drawn to sport. It was either sport nutrition or paediatrics.

I was lucky enough I got an internship with Jennifer Gibson (Jen, who is now my good friend and business partner) and ended up getting a full-time job right out of internship. This full-time position in sport was maybe the second of its kind in Canada at the time. One thing led to another; I worked in Olympic sport for a while and then got bored with a stunted scope of practice. A dietetic education and the IOC course limited the impactful and innovative support I could contribute to gold medal potential in Olympic sport. I could really see that in the Canadian Olympic system: the level of education that practitioners as nutritionists or dietitians had across the country was not really cutting edge and the level of winning Olympic medals. I needed to get more physiology. I needed to figure out how to understand human systems more and really think like a researcher and think outside the box so that I could do more than just help with nutrition. I wanted to be innovative and confident that I'm contributing to improved performance and improved health for athletes. This would also help keep my attention. I get bored easily. Jen and I joke. She calls herself ADD and I'm the ADHD one and we fully are. It's hilarious. But we get it done. We get the job done.

I ended up in Australia in Tasmania, which contrary to popular belief is not in Africa, which I initially thought when my husband brought this job posting to me. We took a job in Tasmania, a far island on the other side of the world. To sweeten the deal I was offered a great funded PhD position. Trent Stellingwerff stayed on as a PhD supervisor and I was able to shape a very cool collaboration with the Canadian Sport Institute Pacific. My heart is very much in Canadian Olympic Sport. The Tassie move proved to continue to open up interesting doors. I got closer to the Australian Institute of Sport, which at the time was *the* hub of sport science and sport nutrition applied research. My PhD work connected me with the amazing gastroenterology and nutrition group at Monash, which was just a quick puddle jump across the water. The connection to that group ended up being integral to shaping the second part of my PhD work in gluten-free diets and FODMAPS in athletes. You see these PhD analogy diagrams, where a tiny, almost invisible dot is within a much larger circle; the circle is the world and the dot is the impact of your research. Given the opportunities created I actually feel like my PhD work is represented by a slightly larger dot, just a little bit larger, because it is really cool when your research actually impacts and shapes sport nutrition approaches for performance dietitians moving forward.

We stayed in Tasmania for 3.5 years and like any early career academic, I got a job offer to come back to North America. My husband would have happily stayed on the island for the rest of his natural born life. But we missed skiing and Australia seemed even further from family (and good skiing) after having a kid. The job offer was with the University of California, Davis, and I knew Dr. Keith Baar there. It all panned out smoothly. To make a short story even shorter, I walked into Keith's office, and he was like, "Hey, I have this postdoc opportunity with GSSI, do you want it?"

People would fight tooth and nail for a position in the Baar lab. I didn't really know what I wanted to do when we moved back to the US. It is the land of opportunity and again, that was another reason we left Tasmania. In some ways, you're a fish in a small pond in Australia, where in the US you're in a huge pond and there are a ton of skills you get to learn to navigate the big pond. So, postdoc, OK, sure, that sounds cool, I'm just finishing up my PhD, I'll do some more research. I ended up staying there for four and a half years and then working with two of the NBA teams locally and then also overseas with World Tour cycling at the same time. Lots, lots of different positions, shuffling and negotiating time and contracts all the time. I stayed at the university till COVID and then I left the university because human research was kind of shut down there and I was at a point too where I wanted to become more entrepreneurial and I wanted to also live in the mountains.

I remember being surprised when as a postdoc at UC Davis I was not handed a new laptop or office space. At UTAS I was handed two brand-new Macs, top of the line ergo desk, along with assessment and fitting. Here is what the big pond is like and I went to IKEA, bought my own desk and found a place to set it up in the building. Based on my observations, many students coming from Australia or other countries where the academic system is set up and funded differently become livid with entitlement. Being a mature student I still have the upbringing to expect nothing to be handed to you and that no one owes you anything. The US student entitlement culture is shocking in this generation and in a big pond you don't waste your time whingeing about how long it takes your supervisor to return your email. I am married to a hardcore academic, my husband "the professor". Academic pressure is intense; as a student, PhD student or post doc, it is important wto maintain appreciation and gratitude to everyone who has mentored you and pay it forward. Even though I cried from being overwhelmed after my first lab meeting in the Baar lab the challenge of diving into a molecular physiology lab was so rewarding. My only regret was trying to work too many different positions while working in the lab. I was never fully where my feet were. Saying "no" to opportunities to work with the world's best athletes/sport scientists is something I am lacking proficiency in.

We spent almost every spare minute we could in Tahoe and ended up lucking out with buying a condo right on Donner Lake. Like any recent story... and then COVID hit. It turned out okay and we kind of just didn't leave. Then COVID kept going so we crafted our life around it. I ended up taking a remote job with Science in Sport in the UK and that was a decent fit for home-schooling. I learned a lot about a new industry and now I am grateful for having every area of sport nutrition covered in terms of:

1. Research (and am still involved in research in less hands-on ways)
2. Practice in elite sport in Europe, US, Australia and Canada and between Olympic, professional, and collegiate
3. Industry

Having experience in what I call "*the triad*" of sport nutrition has given me the confidence to go out on my own and make the entrepreneurial jump. To live in California and a sought-after destination ski town you need to find ways to bulk up the bank account.

I believe that people come in/out of your life at the right times. Jen Gibson, my first sport nutrition mentor during my dietetics internship, reconnected and we were at a parallel point in our lives. One might call it various states of a mid-life crisis. We'd reached a lot of summits physically and metaphorically. We'd done a lot of stuff in our careers, that a lot of people only dream of, and with our Dr. Google-diagnosed ADD and ADHD (joking) we were not happy doing the same job, different team. An email and phone call later we had an LLC, a business model and we ran our first Elite Ops Performance Nutrition course. Purpose was found in investing in the next generation of practitioners and in the US training and education to authentically work in in elite sport is dismal.

I'll be honest, sport nutrition education in the US is antiquated. I maintain that there is sport nutrition and performance nutrition. With the new company, Performance Nutrition Professionals (PNP), we developed this Lab2Life format and are really training practitioners how to work in elite sport. This is the stuff we learned with a cumulative 30+ years of practice, across >24 sports. It's the stuff you don't know you don't know and you can't learn anywhere else. Slowly, but I think we're kind of changing the landscape in the US, which is a very different landscape in sport nutrition than the UK, Canada and Australia. The US sport RD culture can still be a bit undercutting and with PNP we get to challenge this; we are reshaping how professionals uplift the profession by creating this collaborative community of practitioners, giving what we know and also showing our vulnerability. It makes the course experience very real and everyone leaves being friends and for some, apparently, is "a life changing experience", which we did not anticipate.

**That's an interesting background. One thing that I picked up on is not only the experience that you've got, but it's what I'd like to call the craft knowledge of being in at the deep end, in at the trenches of those multiple disciplines within your triad that you explained. If I asked you to reflect on now, how and when did you first get involved in nutrition?**

**Dana:** When I was working in Costa Rica we brought our food to these remote locations, and we'd have bags of flour and quinoa. We didn't have a tonne of food. There was some fresh fruit and vegetables, but it was every third or fourth day and you're feeding a group and so you only have a certain portion. I didn't know much about nutrition when I was 17; all I had done was figure skating. I got kind of fat when I was in Costa Rica the first time. I was eating fried empanadas every day and it's a sense of food scarcity that I've never been used to. I like food. I'm Polish; we like food. When you're living remotely, you don't have mirrors, you don't have scales. I had no idea that I had put on a solid 15 pounds in a couple months. I went back home, and I was like, oh, that happened.

So I had to learn about nutrition which I didn't really know. I was still a teenager, still a kid, really. I didn't really know a tonne about nutrition. So I started learning about it and it was interesting to me how quickly what you put in your body could influence your body in that way. Then working in the outdoor industry, also just the impact of nutrition on brain function and risk assessment and cognitive function, decision making, tiredness. You're putting in long days in the field and I think that the interaction of nutrition on all of those led me into this interest in the nutrition space, and I'd always been involved in sport in one way or another. But sport nutrition was also just cool at that time. It was the place where it was the hardest to get a job. So then I was drawn to getting a job in that space.

**I think I know the answer to this one, but who are your mentors in life and why?**

**Dana:** Well, Jen Gibson definitely and Trent Stellingwerff. He's been an amazing mentor. He's always the guy who's there for you. If there's someone I really want to pay back, it's Trent. He's done so much for my career. Then also Scott Livingston; he is somebody I worked with a bit in Olympic sport in some specialised projects and he's an athletic trainer by trade, also strength and conditioning, and has started this Leave Your Mark podcast and group and he's running this mentorship programme for people like myself who are at transition points in their career, have worked in sport, elite sport or various iterations of that and really need a mentor process that understands the mindset of people who work in elite sport and also just the identity and the ego associated with it. So the psychology of that person and then also the nuances of working in elite sport, like how that affects your life. If you had a regular career mentor or life coach,

I don't think they would get that part of working in elite sport of what it means to your life and how you balance everything. It's not a normal job and also the psyche associated with it, there's an ego associated with it, and when you decide to step away from elite sport or step away from working full time in it, you have to deal with letting part of your identity go, and that that's been huge for me and Scott's been amazing through that process. I'm probably happier now with the way I work in sport than I've ever been in my whole career, so I think I developed through that. I've really learned there are lots of different ways you can create a career in professional sport. You've just got to think outside the box and you have to put the hours in. You've got to put the time in early on when you don't have a family and you're looking to build up your experience, but you don't have to do that your entire life.

**Yeah, yeah. 100% agree and it's exactly where I am at now with the massive family chapter of having a daughter and all I want to do is spend time at home. Do you know what I mean?**

**So what has been a standout moment in your career so far?**

**Dana:** Yeah, there've definitely been a few. I think one of them is there are the bigwigs, the big movers and shakers in our industry, who've been around my whole career like Louise Burke, Stuart Phillips, Trent, and being on panels with them and at ACSM or GSSI, basically making it to that level… I don't like to have this hierarchy thing but those are the people that have been around. They have shaped what performance nutrition is to this date and to be able to be invited to speak on panels with those people has probably been a standout moment in my career. I've worked hard and it's paid off and here are some of the rewards. I think that's probably been one of the standout moments for sure.

**Yeah, that's amazing, and anything from within sport itself? In terms of you've won the championship or an athlete did something big?**

**Dana:** You know what, it's funny, even though I've been with the Golden State Warriors through two championships, as a consultant I really don't feel like it's even in part my win to celebrate. I'm usually not on site for championship games, so I don't feel celebrating the win the same way as the full-time staff who live and breathe their jobs. I celebrate and honour their tireless work. I did get a cool W jersey with my name on it. Everyone asks, "Did you get a ring?" (the ring that the winning team gets).

Olympic sport is where I can comfortably feel like my support was impactful and part of the journey to the podium. Several Canadian Olympic medals stand out and more recently, one of our Canadian speed skaters was able to go home with some bling. I have to be careful about confidentiality, but in the last year of the squad we worked together and I can confidently say her mindset around fuelling and technically nutrition strategy was one of the deciding factors getting her on the podium, more than once. That was a more recent standout moment.

A more personal moment was riding through the Rhone Alps with Chris Froome. Holy crap, how did I get here. At a training camp where my sole purpose was to ensure we were doing everything to get him into Tour de France shape. Riding through what I consider heaven on earth with a four-time TdF winner. Unfortunately after his crash he hasn't been able to perform at that level again, yet...

**That's amazing. For you, what is an influential factor as to why you're successful in your career? Because you are successful, you know, to be invited onto round tables with the people that you've mentioned.**

**Dana:** Yeah, I think historically it was a tireless work ethic. I don't work as hard anymore as I have got a kid. I don't work till I fall asleep every single night. But earlier in my career I had a tireless work ethic. I would work my ass off night and day. There was never a night I wasn't working after dinner. I would go ski touring in university and bring textbooks with me. You go ski touring as long as possible but I would bring chemistry textbooks with me because I had an exam Monday – stupid.

So I think definitely the tireless effort. The drive for me was always actually the mindset of I was never good enough. There was always something else I wanted to achieve and that had its pros and cons. It keeps you going and it keeps you striving to learn more and do different things and think outside the box. But it doesn't allow you to celebrate your accomplishments either. So I think earlier in my career that was maybe a good thing because I just always kept going. But now, I'm able to sit back and appreciate what I've done and sit in that glory for a bit. So one would be a tireless work ethic.

Two would be just international experience. You just get so much more exposure to the different ways people work. So I think having an international mindset and an international exposure were definitely key to my success because not everything's happening in your country or your circle of practitioners, or your professional governing body. Look outside of that. If I'm doing the same thing day to day, I just get bored easily, so that you're always looking for what's next. I've also been lucky enough to have some great people come into my life that have opened my eyes to what's available in the sport world and what you need to do to get there. I wanted to be the best in the world or one of the best in the world and you need to do research. You need to have practice in a tonne of different areas. You need to have a clinical background. You need to have management skills and I think all of those have helped with some of those successes as well. Honestly, my husband too, he's a rock. He supports me in anything. He's a rock and I'm surprised he's still with me.

**What's been one of your biggest challenges in your career so far? Because it's not always a straight line.**

**Dana:** I think letting my ego go. I say I've let it go, but I'm not sure I have because I still have my name attached to a professional team. Would I be OK if that stopped tomorrow? I might take a little bit of time to get over it. But I've done enough in my career that I have the confidence now I think that I am good at what I do. I still need to keep learning though. I don't want to sit back and be like I've done all this, I'm good to go for another few years and then I'll retire. No, I still have 20 years left of work, scary as it is. So I think that probably the biggest challenge is letting my ego go and being comfortable with the fact it's pro sport; you might get fired the next day. How is that going to affect you? Are you going to be a depressed mess? Or have you thought through those scenarios already and done enough of what I call the mental hygiene to be able to work through those challenges?

You get some tough people to work with in pro sport and your ego is going to get bruised and you're going to not be sure if you're going to have a job tomorrow in some cases. I think just doing the mental work and the mental hygiene to not let your ego attach to your job and your identity to attach to your job too much early on is probably what I'd advise younger practitioners. Be your own person outside of your job; try to keep that as separate as you can.

**Yeah. So difficult when the hours of sport can be so long and you end up spending more time with your colleagues at work than you do with friends and family, don't you?**

**Dana:** Yeah, in a way you choose your colleagues at work. You choose your sport to a certain extent, and if you have a great franchise like the Warriors which are a fantastic group to work for... the culture there is incredibly well developed; it's a great culture. I've worked at a couple NBA franchises and they're all different. I've been lucky enough to get connected with a really good franchise and that's one that in a way you choose and that's like a family and the colleagues that you choose, where with your own family, you don't always choose them.

I think there's also a lot of guilt associated with being super married to your job and spending a lot of time there.

There are certain points in your career that you need to do that if you want to have a really, vibrant, successful long-term career in elite sport; you need to put the hours in early on. You're going to be there; they are going to be your family for a while. But just do that that mental work early on, and still keep part of your life separate from the facility and the team.

**Yeah, for sure. Linked into that, what characteristics do you think people need to work on or research in sport nutrition?**

**Dana:** I think you need to be humble and really realise there's a lot you don't know and just be super curious and that's one thing that's been pretty influential for me is I've always been really curious about mechanisms. It's really easy to get this prescription from Instagram and that's one thing that Jen and my company are trying to pull back a bit from, this prescriptive nutrition mentality of younger practitioners who can just go on Instagram and just be like "Oh, here's a protocol for beta alanine, here you go" and not really understand the mechanisms, not understand the sport, that prescription is not going to work for this characteristic. We don't use beta alanine with this typical protocol in the NBA. There are so many other factors that you need to be able to analyse and you need to know these nuances, so I think, yeah, I've always been very curious and very much need to understand the mechanisms for anything related to nutrition.

I want to understand how that affects different pathways so I can make a really educated decision on how to use certain strategies. So definitely that curious mind and humility for sure. Also just having the interpersonal skills; being an outward bound instructor and working at summer camps when I was younger pretty well developed my interpersonal skills. I can work in groups pretty well and I can read people and know when to turn on certain aspects of my personality to work with the team.

So a strong interpersonal skill set is also really important for working in sport as well as research. It's funny, we have a tenant living at our house in Davis and him and I joke and no offence to career students, but we always joke about the lack of social skills that career students like postdocs have.

They've never left school and they postdoc for, like, 20 years. We always joke about how socially inept they are. I was talking to my husband and I'm like is this just my perception, but he's like no. It makes sense if you've just seen academia your whole life; that's your world. You become a bit socially inept and it made me feel sorry for a lot of people. But it brought to light how these super-smart researchers that we look up to in a way, they don't work in sport and just having quite a few years having that academic persona as well as having one foot in sport really allowed me to balance things. I was able to ask the questions on both ends as I developed a research question and worked through a study and then also as we worked through new strategies for a team, having that sort of leading edge research going on the side with injury stuff with NBA, that's super-pertinent. So having both of those happening at the same time allowed me to be at the leading edge on both sides, where I could take in real practical experience and then also laboratory stuff and be able to use it right away because I was physically in both locations at the same time.

**Yeah, class. What would be your recommendations to a new student entering the industry now?**

**Dana:** One of the things I would say is probably any entitlement you think you have, lose it – you are not owed anything. I do see a different mindset with the newer generation and people. I mean, our parents probably said that about us. But I would say be humble, take the mindset that you're not entitled to anything, you have to work for it. No one owes you anything and be inquisitive and get international experience if you can. Think outside the box would probably be another one. Really think outside the box because if you want to be an innovative practitioner or researcher or both, you need to have that mindset that you're going to not do what's already been done. You're going to try to ask those questions about what's not been done or why are things not being done, or why is it not? Why is it this way? But why is it not doing being done this way? So I think definitely be very inquisitive. Inquisitive to your approaches, curious, put in the hard work, lose the entitlement. Create your own path for sure. Sometimes we have this pure academic path, that we think we need to go into university after we've done high school. If you're not ready for it or you want to do something else first, really do your own self-discovery and your own path and I think you'd be much happier.

**Everyone's got their own journey. Are there any areas on nutrition courses that are not currently taught at all, which you think would be good to learn?**

**Dana:** I think newer practitioners or students looking to come into the industry should be prepared to do research, get involved in research early, like during your undergrad, if you can volunteer for being a subject, if you can volunteer in a lab, that is going to get you so much valuable experience.

Yeah, it sucks entering Excel numbers, it sucks holding a pen or measuring something for hours. But you've got to put in the time. I remember I had a student once who was like I've done my undergrad, I never expected to be recording numbers for four hours. I was like, I didn't expect to be cooking 500 meals during my PhD. Guess what I did? I cooked 500 meals and measured the gluten content in it. You always have to be able to do everything and I think you have to learn how to do everything if you want to go into research or practice or anything or you want to be innovative, you've got to learn how to do every part of that job. There's never any part of a team that is too small for you to do or too menial of a task for you to do. You've gotta buy the toilet paper; you've gotta wipe asses sometimes too. Just being willing to do some of those small jobs and learn from them. Get involved in research as much as you can. If you really want to excel in the performance nutrition or sport industry, you're probably going to have to have an advanced degree of some sort or some combination, and then courses that I didn't get that I wish I got, were much more physiology, exercise physiology, rehab. A lot of what we do is keeping athletes healthy ready to return to play, statistics, research skills and management and leadership skills. There are a lot of courses where students don't get an opportunity to learn through a traditional academic programme. With all the online learning, there are lots of opportunities to get some of these skills elsewhere. But then also think outside of the box of where you can get those skills, like I mentioned the outdoor industry. There are lots of opportunities to do outdoor programmes where you don't have to sit in front of a computer to get these skills, go do it without.

**Where do you think the future of nutrition will be in five years' time?**

**Dana:** Yeah, I think it's exciting actually. We have a lot of really talented nutritionists that are getting more and more skilled worldwide. The research and the practitioners that are coming out of LJMU with incredible skill sets, straight out of university and yeah, they're still gonna need to get the experience. But I think we're going to have more practitioners that are specialised, like you might be specialised in just altitude nutrition. So you might be somebody that a cycling team brings in for certain blocks and certain expertise. My vision of what it is going to look like is that every professional and Olympic team will have a high level, well, at least one high level performance nutritionist integrated into the team and then I see that split into two where we're going to have more of the food service specialisation. So food service and that whole piece is going to be more performance oriented and have a practitioner or practitioners that are more in the food service, performance fuelling space and then more of the innovation and research, physiology space crossover. So ideally every team has at least two people to cover each of those core areas and then practitioners who are specialised. It could be blood glucose stuff with the whole continuous glucose monitoring stuff we're doing now; it could be altitude. It might be low energy availability. What are the priorities or the key performance priorities or key issues that you see in certain sports and certain teams and then bring in experts for certain blocks such as the Olympic cycle. So I see that specialisation and then I see within a team a continual performance nutrition team of at least two or more people.

**Yeah. Yeah. Interesting. I like that. The final three questions are probably more rapid fire. Is there a book that you would recommend right now?**

**Dana:** *The Four Agreements*, hands down. It's a simple read, but the messages in there, I always operate by them, and the biggest one in that book is never take anything personally. Sport can be hard; you can take losses personally. You can take comments from a coach personally. You can take an athlete's bad day personally. If you did all of that, you'd be miserable and so really never take anything personally is the one core message from that book. You could always use Blinkist too for any books. Blinkist is an app that summarises books quickly. I was addicted to it for a while.

**What key principles do you follow every day?**

**Dana:** I always write down and I used to always work with a to-do list but I would never get through them and that was something I worked a lot on the last year and a half with Scott [Livingston] on his mentorship programme. I always had way too much on my list to do; we would go through these 90-day intentions and I would have these lists in every block and he's like, are you getting that done?

I was like, either I'll kill myself getting them done or I won't get them done. So I've moved away from a to-do list to more intention lists, so I have four categories. One is the career so work, relationships, health and spirit, and I have my intentions for the day. So it's more about intentional living and priorities in each of those categories. I'll only put two or three in each rather than the 10 that I used to have. So I'm trying not to overcommit myself and then feel like I failed today because I didn't get that stuff done, so really being realistic about my time.

With my cell phone and media being away from family time, I don't just pull my phone out first thing in the morning. I don't pull it out until I start my work day and at night too, same thing. I don't need to have it out at night, so I'm just really keeping media separate and work separate from family time. I think another principle that a lot of people struggle with is use of social media; it does have a place. It can be used really well but I'm very intentional with my use of social media. It's either used for work or for some piece of research.

If something pops up in my email, like somebody sharing a research study that interests me, I don't just go on it to look; I'm very intentional. With social media use, I think we waste a lot of time and I'll always do some checks when I feel like I'm not operating super efficiently, to see I'm just wasting time or f***ing around. I will do a check of, hey, what am I doing each 15 minutes of the day to then re-evaluate how I'm working or what's not going well. What am I not operating with, am I f***ing away three hours of the day, just trying to figure out what I'm going to do or on social media or answering emails that aren't a priority? So I'll always do a bit of an evaluation of how I'm using my time so that I'm using it more efficiently and not wasting it with stuff that's not important. So really, it's just a very prioritised based way of operating. I always ask myself, when I'm responding to something, do I need to do this right now or can it wait? Most of the time it can wait and even emails, we get caught up in emails, like it's got to be answered. I'll just answer these 20 emails and then half your day's gone. Whereas the shit that I need to get done that day, that doesn't get done because I've just done the easy thing which is do what's immediately in front of me. So just being very priority driven and reflective on what I'm doing each day and how I'm using my time.

**Yeah, that's class. There's an app that I've been using recently called TickTick and have you heard of The Eisenhower Matrix? That's been really effective for me just to prioritise. I can get a lot of items that need doing and then I can categorise them into different quadrants and then I can put a date and a time that they need to be done by and then it basically prioritises your week and month for you.**

**Dana:** Ohh, I'm totally gonna check that out. Anything that saves me time from writing that out is good. Any accountability mechanism is definitely helpful for me. Yeah, because you're self-employed it's sometimes easy just to say I'll do it tomorrow; no one is going to fire me.

**Oh yeah, that's it. Finally, last question, in your eyes, what makes a successful performance nutritionist?**

**Dana:** I think you've gotta be a people person. You've gotta have a dynamic personality. You need to be very self-aware and that's on every level of yourself. Then also how you interact with athletes and within a group. Just being a reflective person who's looking to improve and looking to get better at every facet of your life. You need to be somewhat of a leader for sure because a lot of times performance nutrition is a newer position in a team.

You're not going to have somebody tell you how to do your job. No one really knows what you do so you do have to be a leader and an innovative thinker. I think you have to be pretty humble and it's easy to sometimes get a bit of an ego that you're the performance nutritionist for this team, but you just stay humble because you might not be tomorrow. I think how you measure success also changes over your career. What I would have said 10 years ago when I would have viewed myself as a successful practitioner would have definitely been different than what I would say now, as more of a mature practitioner. Ten years ago as a younger practitioner, I would have said you've gotta be a hard worker, you've got to be on top of research, you've got to be always willing to be available for your team. I do still think that is necessary to be a successful practitioner from a technical perspective. Then there's the soft skills area as well that needs to be equally as developed to be a successful performance nutritionist. So your technical skills, your soft skills, and bringing those together into that person, into that leader who's managing the performance nutrition programme, is what I think you need to be successful in any of those positions.

**That's golden. Absolutely golden. So that draws the interview to an end.**

## JAMES'S THOUGHTS

Although Dana and I have very different lives and career paths, an area we connected on straight away was the travelling and a few years of global experience first, before committing to study in higher education.

A particular point of this interview which stands out was when Dana said: *"Saying 'no' to opportunities to work with the world's best athletes/ sport scientists is something I am lacking proficiency in."* I can appreciate what she is saying here as I have found myself in these situations before. As you get older, you learn to say no more but it can be tempting as a young student, early career researcher or practitioner to say yes to everything! It is a fine balance!

I love how Dana speaks about any entitlement you think you have, lose it now! Also, just be curious and appreciate that there is a lot you do not know, and will never know, but that's life!

Finally, again another practitioner talking about how important it is to be a people person, be dynamic and build better relationships with all those people around you.

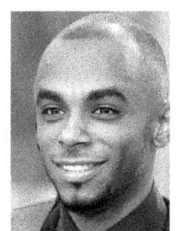

# CHAPTER 10:
## MOHAMED SAAD

Mohamed is the founder of Arab Academy for Sports Nutrition and product expert consultant for Red Bull in the Middle East. He has previous experience as the head of nutrition and weight cut specialist with KHK Sports and sports performance lab specialist with the Bahrain Olympic Committee.

I have never met Mohamed in person but remember reading his Nutrition X article about Ramadan and enjoying what he wrote. He has a diploma from the Institute of Performance Nutrition and an MSc from Middlesex University.

You can follow Mohamed on:
Twitter @mohamedsaadbh
Instagram @mohamedsaadbh

**So to kick this off, give us a quick introduction as to who you are and what your background is.**

**Mohamed:** My name is Mohamed, Mohamed Saad, I'm Bahraini and based in Bahrain as well. To be honest, my background wasn't in nutrition. I grew up as a kid that loves sports, I did a lot of kinds of sports. Most of them are martial arts, taekwondo, capoeira, Muay Thai, mixed martial arts; they are the sports that I love most and also bodybuilding. I love the physique type of sport as well. From there, I loved learning how I develop my body, how I enhance my performance, but I didn't know anything about nutrition back then. Even just the basics, what is protein? What are carbs? Fats? That's it. From there, I started to try to learn by myself, but I didn't get through anything. I just started reading through bodybuilding.com trying to learn about supplements, nutrition, but there wasn't solid knowledge there.

So after that, when I graduated from high school, I did my undergraduate in international logistics management. When I did my bachelor's degree, I finished and I started to do postgraduate certificates like the IOPN with Laurent Bannock back then in 2014, I believe. From there, I've taken it from the postgraduate diploma to the master's degree. I did my master's degree in sports nutrition, at Middlesex University in London, where I did my last academic studying.

**Can you paint the picture for me and maybe some others, of what does the sports nutrition arena look like in Bahrain?**

**Mohamed:** Ah, man, I struggled a lot to try to convince the authorities in Bahrain about sports nutrition. Even the athletes, they know nothing. It's like you started from scratch. I did everything from scratch. So to be honest, when I started, nothing was there. All they know is what bodybuilding says, the things happening in the bodybuilding industry, other than that nothing. Talking about football, talk about any type of endurance athletes, they have no knowledge of nutrition. They just do what they believe is right to be done based on what they heard from their coaches. But are there any sports nutritionists in the field in Bahrain? Unfortunately not. That's when I started but now it's starting to develop more and more. I think we're still not there but we are pushing hard to get it there since the time I have finished my studying.

**So in regard to nutrition, you obviously mentioned your background wasn't in nutrition. You then did the IOPN and then your master's at Middlesex. When did you first get involved in applied nutrition as a performance nutritionist with an athlete or with a team?**

**Mohamed:** Let me tell you, there was a period which was missing between when I started to love nutrition and when I started to apply it. I was doing a sport called parkour and I had a team called Bahrain Parkour, which is the first team of parkour and free running in Bahrain. So back then in 2010, I got interviewed by Bahrain TV, which is our national television. When I was done with the interview, I got called by one of the managers at the TV channel. He told me that I like the way you speak, and I want you to work with us. I said I have nothing to do with TV; I didn't study media, nothing, and he said no problem, we'll teach you, we like your character. I said, okay, no problem and then I started from there as a TV presenter. The supervisor of the TV told me: we want to do a nutrition segment which is live, and I want you to run it and you just interview dietitians, and I said no problem.

Back then I started to prepare for the segments; I was doing a lot of reading and I thought this is interesting, I need to get more involved in that. So this period when I was in the TV was when I fell in love with nutrition, especially sports nutrition, because I love sports. So I wanted something related to sports. So I started to develop that. At the same time I was doing my IOPN and when I finished it, I got a call from one of the football coaches, he's a good friend, he told me, I believe in what you do. We don't have a sports nutritionist but I want you to be involved with us and the national team. I'm fighting for it but they are saying it's not necessary. Why do we need a nutritionist? What value will he add? I didn't blame them because they don't have the knowledge. They don't know anything about that. They believe that it all comes from the coach; he does everything. So I told him no problem, I'll work for free. I don't want any money. I just want to prove that it is important to get a nutritionist.

So in 2016, I worked with the Bahrain U19 national football team, and we worked for the Asian Cup. The feedback that I got from the coach, the feedback I got from the athletes was phenomenal. To be honest, many of them said we didn't feel we could even finish the first half due to lack of energy, but now we can finish the full match with full energy. So we can definitely feel what nutrition does, we feel better, our recovery is much better.

Even the physical coach said the nutrition that you give them, even their physique has become much better. So the feedback that I got was amazing, and then they reported it to the Bahrain Football Association. The Federation said wow, this is something interesting and we have to consider it in the future. So that was the first time I applied nutrition in the field. At that time, also, the Federation wrote an article about me and the newspaper said, the first nutritionist in the history of Bahrain to be with our national team. So that was amazing, to be honest, to experience. Since then, I finished with the football team when we didn't make it to the Asian Cup. But since I finished with them, I started to work with the MMA. From here I started to work with different sports. I work with individual athletes across 20 different sports so I have worked with many athletes since my first experience with the football team back in 2016.

**Amazing. That was a really, really good story. Really nice to hear that. In regard to mentors in your life, who have your mentors been and why have they been important for you?**

**Mohamed:** Yeah. Well, the first mentor that I knew was Laurent Bannock. I remember back then, when I did my IOPN, I remember Laurent had a course like three or four days in his Guru Performance Institute in London. I didn't have the money but I wanted to travel, I wanted to learn, so I sold many things I have in my house just to make the money to travel there. So I travelled to London and I met him in person and I told him I'm keen to learn, I'm hungry for knowledge. That's why I came all the way from Bahrain to be here. All of the other guys were there from UK, nobody had travelled from other countries, so he really appreciated what I did, and that showed him how much I wanted to learn. So he taught me a lot of things; I learned a lot from Laurent. Laurent was my first mentor; he was really generous in the information that he gave me. He shifted my career in the way that he helped me.

Also another person who I really look up to is Graeme Close; he is a good friend. To be honest, I learned a lot from him. He was always supporting me. I also did an article with him about Ramadan. That was two years ago and since then my relationship with Graeme has been amazing and still is amazing, now also with Laurent too, so Laurent and Graeme, both of them. They were the mentors that I had, the people that I was looking up to. So yeah, they have added a lot of value to my career.

**Yeah, the Nutrition X article is a really good one, actually. It's one that I've read a few times because it's an area that I just don't know enough about, to be honest, and a lot of nutritionists in England would not have a clue about that area of nutrition. So yeah, a very valuable tool that. So in your career so far, what would you say has been a standout moment for you?**

**Mohamed:** Since I finished with the football team and I shifted to the MMA, mixed martial arts, I have been working with two teams, one team called Khaled bin Hamad Al Khalifa (KHK) MMA and our national MMA team. KHK MMA is a mixture of amateur and professional MMA fighters. When I started to work with MMA fighters in different competitions, regionally and internationally, we did the Europe competition, Asian, African Open, all around the world. But the moment that we did the World Championship, we won it, and Bahrain had the title and was ranked number one, man, I just can't tell you how that feels.

I have worked with these guys from zero. They were making a lot of mistakes. MMA fighters do weight cuts, they eat rubbish food, they don't know what to do. I've started to help them to put everything in its place and do the weight making in the right scenario and they felt much better. Even the coach was telling me, I can see the recovery, how they are doing. So it felt nice to know that some of my work assisted the team to become the world champions, you know.

So that was one of the best moments in my career and we made it four times; four times in a row we were the world champions. We beat everyone and that was amazing. We are now ranked number one as a national team in the world in IMMAF, which is the International Mixed Martial Arts Federation. We made more than 100 medals; we have the top male and female fighters in the world in amateurs. That's amazing to be part of this achievement.

**And what's the population of Bahrain?**

**Mohamed:** It's 1.7 million, so when you compare that to the USA alone, a World Champion is pretty special, right?

MMA to be honest is a new sport in Bahrain. How it was developed, His Highness Sheikh Khalid bin Hamad, who is the President of the Bahrain Olympic Committee, he loved MMA and started to practise it and he said, you know what, I'll do my team which is called KHK, which is Khalid bin Hamad Al Khalifa's.

So he created the KHK MMA team and he said, okay, I'll sponsor athletes, I'll do everything they need. He built a big place for MMA. In 2015 when I joined, that was the first year ever and he brought legends like Khabib Nurmagomedov; he was with us in the team for like a year and a half and then he left. Also Islam Makhachev who is his mate; we have also our head coach who is a tremendous athlete and unbeatable fighter. His name is Eldar Eldarov and he is the one who made our team the best in the world. So we started from zero with the support of His Highness and we pushed so hard until they became the world champions. So it needs a lot of effort, money and a lot of things to prepare a team that is a world class team.

**That's brilliant. So with where you've come from, and then doing the nutrition in 2014/2015 to where you are now, what do you think is the influential factor that you've got, that's allowed you to be successful in your career so far?**

**Mohamed:** Okay, do you mean the thing that helped me in general or something that I own that helped me in my personality? What do you mean, exactly?

**Yeah, I would say in general, because we will discuss your traits later.**

**Mohamed:** To be honest, I would say, social media is power. If I don't know you, I will not do business with you. If I'm not there, showing the knowledge that I have, I have shared what I do, I would have done none of this; how I got all of these was because I was there showing people the knowledge, I was telling them what sports nutrition is and how important it is.

So athletes started to follow me, and they started to listen, from there, they believed in that. So that opened a big door for me. That's why I believe now that every nutritionist should be on social media, not just social media posting just every couple of days or every couple of weeks; you have to be there all the time. Why? Because you need to show yourself to everyone. So everyone knows you; if everyone knows you, everyone will work with you. So to be honest, a big part of my success, I will say most of it, was through social media because people supported me there; they will try to share the things that I post. I reach different countries all over, the Arabic speakers, and people started to invite me to be a speaker at their conferences, to look after their athletes. So the most influential factor that turned my career into a success or so is social media. Social media is power.

**I would agree. And it still baffles me, years ago, to advertise globally would have cost millions. Whereas now because of LinkedIn, Instagram, Twitter, TikTok, whatever, you've got the ability to go global and it doesn't cost a penny.**

**Mohamed:** Exactly. It's so easy. I would say now, if you compare nowadays with 20/30 years ago, success is quicker because now you can reach everyone easily. You don't have to travel, you don't have to call, you don't have to do this and that. You just have the power of your phone and your brain. That's it. And you can just be there everywhere. So yeah, I believe social media is a big part of many people's success nowadays. Because the more people that know you, the more you will have opportunities to reach and achieve.

**Yeah. What's been the biggest challenge of your career so far?**

**Mohamed:** Let me tell you the first one. I remember when I started nutrition. I went to the Athletics Federation in Bahrain and nobody knew me at that time. I told them I want to meet the president of the Federation, and they asked me what do you want? Are you an athlete? No. Why do you want to meet him? I just want to tell him something that's important to consider for the athletes. Okay, no problem. They told him and he said, let him in. I told him my name is Mohamed, I am studying nutrition and I believe nutrition is a big factor. He was looking at me and he's smiling like, okay. I told him, I want to work with you guys for free. I'm giving all my time for you guys just for free. I want you to see; I want you to try it. He was like, um, well, we don't have much time now. But we'll try to call you later on, leave your number. Nobody even called me though. So this was the first step where I felt there's a big struggle to convince the authorities in Bahrain about nutrition.

Step by step I tried my best through social media and they started to see, and then when I worked with the football national team, they started to listen to what athletes have started to say. After all of this, I remember this is one of the best moments I had in my lifetime, His Highness Sheikh Nasser bin Hamad, who is the son of the king, he was following me on Instagram and I was like, wow, he's following me and then they told me he wants to meet you. So I went there. I just couldn't believe that; he's someone everyone looks up to. He is the son of the king.

He told me, Mohamed, I've heard a lot of great things of you, I have seen your social media. He was a triathlete and he said, I want you to be my nutritionist for triathlon. I was like, that's an honour, I will do it. So for seven years, I worked with His Highness to be his nutritionist. He was so happy about the results. Then he said, I'll help you. If you want to study, if you want to do anything, I'll support you. So Him, and His Highness Sheikh Khalid bin Hamad Al Khalifa, both of them supported me to do my master's degree and to do my studies; if I needed anything related to the field of nutrition, there was a lot of support from their side.

Then, whenever I tell His Highness that this sport needs some nutrition, this sport needs it too, he listens and he said, yes, I agree. So from that moment, His Highness started to tell the authorities in Bahrain, listen to Mohamed, take from him what can benefit you. Now they started to listen, they started to apply and even though we still didn't reach what we really needed to reach they started to listen, they started to call me if there was anything when their athletes had a problem, what we needed to feed them, what should we give them in supplements, which supplement we take. So now I said wow, people have started to believe and started to understand, because I remember one time His Highness posted a picture of me and him on his Instagram, which has hundreds of thousands of followers. He said, Mohamed helped me a lot, he helped me with my nutrition and nutrition is important. So people were like, wow, okay, His Highness is saying that, then we should do that as well, you know. So that was a big boost, to be honest, also, in my career. So at the start of my career it was very hard to convince people; it was struggling to let them understand how valuable nutrition is. But still, there are a couple of people who are in the sport industry who we are still working to convince but it's much better than before.

**That's amazing and the fact that like what you said earlier, this has all really come off you driving your own social media and people seeing it and getting in touch via it. Some might say, oh, that's luck, or you've just been lucky in your career. But the one thing that I'm getting from you is that deep down there's a real drive to go out there and to get the work and to be exposed and be vulnerable because you know that it only takes the one Royal Highness to put a post up and boom, your exposure goes through the roof.**

**Mohamed:** If I wasn't prepared, I wouldn't get it. What is luck? It's the opportunity when it meets preparation. If you have the opportunity if you're not prepared, you cannot do anything and if you're not prepared, and you get the opportunity, what you going to do? You will never know who will see your social media, who will be convinced of the things they listen to, who will call you to come and work with them. I've got a lot of opportunities in my life; I work with people I've never thought I would even come close to. Why, because I put myself there, I pushed myself out and let people know me. So if everyone tried to do that, I think you would get there; just push yourself and keep going.

**So we're beginning to talk about the next question. What characteristics do you think are important to work in the field of performance nutrition?**

**Mohamed:** You should be influential. I think it's very important to know how to talk, how to convince; I don't believe that it's only knowledge that we take in university, it's important to keep an influence on the people around you. Now, if I have a lot of athletes I'm working with in a club or a national team, I'm just doing my job, putting in the supplements, giving them food, preparing the meals with a chef and I'm just doing my job. But how can we influence the athletes, talk to them, speak to them, be close to them? It's really important to me, if you want to be successful, to build the characteristics that you need to be a good performance nutritionist. You have to build your character, you have to build the way you speak, you have to build the way you convince people to work in everything that may help you to reach these people from the inside.

It isn't just about information. Everyone gives information. Why do people love that guy but not that guy? This guy knows how to talk, knows how to convince, he is good with these people and built a relationship with them. So be influential, it's very important to be influential; also, be patient. If you're not patient, it's hard to get there. I believe patience is important, because not everyone has the same level of knowledge. Not everyone has the same level of understanding; I may have 20 different athletes, if I tell them the same information, maybe half of them will get it, half of them will not. So you have to be patient with people; you have to understand people as well.

I really follow something which has really helped me a lot, which is understanding human nature. Everyone is different. Everyone came from a different background. They have had different traumas in their life. So we have to understand and read people; the more we do that I believe the more we will reach out to them, the more we reach them, the more they will believe in us. If they believe in us what will happen? They will talk about us, and if they talk about us, they will bring more people to us and believe in us. So I believe it's really important to be influential, to be patient and to know how to talk with people. This is also plus the knowledge you have.

**What would be your biggest recommendation to your younger self, or aspiring students entering the industry now?**

**Mohamed:** I would say move faster but in what way? If I knew what I knew back then, I would be more successful than now. Why? Because I know I need to be quicker. I had a lot of time when I was just sitting, wasting my time. Sitting in my comfort zone. I just read a bit of the papers, I sat there playing PlayStation, watching movies. But if I had put the real time in, at that time, it would have been a shortcut. Because I believe everyone is working hard. Everyone's working hard but a lot of people are lazy about keeping going. I may read some books. I may read some papers, I'll take a long rest.

Get faster; speed is important. It's really important that you try to push yourself as much as possible, especially if you're young. Let's say you're in your 20s, if you are in your early 20s, it's the base of your future life if you build it well. In our 20s, I believe we want to have fun, we want to enjoy our time. I'm now 36. If I knew what I know now, back then in my 20s, man, my life would be different. I would say, get out of your comfort zone, push yourself hard. The time will come to enjoy your life. Just get there. Let people know you. I know some young guys who are 20/22. Now, man, I really love watching these guys working really hard every day posting on social media to give their clients a point to show people what they have, what they know. So they build their base from a young age. The more you work on that at that time, the faster you will get. So get out of your comfort zone, don't waste your time, move faster. Speed is important to get there and you'll find yourself at the end of the road.

**Yeah, it's such an important point. I've worked with younger nutritionists coming through, you speak to them on the phone, you have dialogues on LinkedIn, and I just get the feeling that unfortunately, we've got a wave of nutritionists coming through, not everyone, but I do think there's a wave that, like what you said, they're just lazy, they just think that they can do the master's and then just get the job without doing anything. I mean, the amount of free work that it sounds like you've done in Bahrain to get where you are, and to get your exposure and to get the experience is insane. It really frustrates me when people think that they can just enter**

our industry, study their undergrad and master's, and then they're going to go and have an amazing career. All they think they have to do is like one picture or share one story; it takes time, it's hard work.

**Mohamed:** Exactly, it's a hard time; you have to put the work in. If you think you will just get your master's degree and get the job and that's it, no, life is much bigger than that. Don't think about it now, think about what is it for me? What should I do next? How can I get bigger? I was speaking earlier to one of my friends; I told him sometimes in life, when we look at things we look at, you know, the horse, when they keep those black things on the sides of their eyes and they just look to the front, we shouldn't keep that, we have to take it off and look around us, then you will find amazing things you love. You can get people to know you more, you get different opportunities. It's not just the job you do as a nutritionist in work like in a club or in a clinic. No, it's not just that, you have a lot of opportunities in life to get there, get connected with people. I believe connection is really important; you have to make it to build a network. Yes, you have to get your network there. As we said earlier, man, the internet is easy. Now I can see this guy. Wow, this guy is smart, I will send him a direct message. Hey, man, my name is blah, blah, blah. And I really like what you do. I want to do something with you. I want to learn from you. I want to do a podcast with you. Whatever it is, even if you message 10 people and one of them replies then that's a win. Instead of sitting down thinking, what do I do today? Well, let me just tweet one tweet, and I'll sleep. Come on, man, work hard, be connected. There's a lot of countries around the world. Get connected to everyone that is in your industry, believe me it helps you somehow and you will get there. So you need to put the work in.

**Is there anything that you didn't learn on the IOPN and the Middlesex master's which has actually been important for you now that you're working full time in nutrition?**

**Mohamed:** I may say that the weight cut and the weight making in MMA was something out of context when it comes to what I've learned. It was a big struggle for me. I had a couple of athletes who would faint and I was like, what should I do, what's happening here? I tried to build up my practice; I did more than a hundred weight cuts with my guys. So I believe there's many things that in practice, may not work as you may read in the books. I believe the context matters because if you read a book or review a study, there's a context for that.

But some people are different. So when you work with athletes in the field, you will see sometimes that's something different than what I've studied, there's something different than what I know. So I have to have this critical thinking and analysing to start to come up with your own tools. That's why you have to build your own tools. Okay, you get some from the knowledge you had in the university or from the courses that you did, and also from the practice you are making with the guys and you bring your own tools that fit your practice. So I believe the experience helps a lot to build these tools. It's a game between knowledge and practice. Bridging the gap between science and practice is really important to make it in this industry.

I learned context from Laurent; I would say context, context and when he says bridging the gap between science and practice, this is really important. You can see now how Laurent influenced me as a mentor; even the things I say are similar. So yeah, it's context, it's how to bridge the gap between science and practice to get there, it's not only about what you read, because if you are just about the science, you'll not get there. You have to have this critical thinking. Be sceptical, but open-minded.

**Yeah. 100%. Where do you think the future of nutrition will be in the next five years? So this question for me has been born out of people like David Dunne, who used to be a nutritionist. He spent 10 years in pro sport, and he's now gone down the technology route in terms of the Hexis app, and you've now got Laurent, who's got his own app. So, where do you think it's going to be in five years' time?**

**Mohamed:** Well, that's a tough question, because it is an endlessly improving, revolutionary industry. What I thought five years ago, again, there was another thing that will come after five years. So it's an endless industry, it's improving every now and then. Always there is something new; sometimes we build our knowledge on something and then we find that it wasn't enough or it wasn't clear, and we try to make new knowledge here. So I think it's a big industry, it's getting there for more improvement, more innovation. But I believe, maybe in the future, we will see more about individualised nutrition in the way of maybe genomics in the future. Still, this area's too early to talk about. But I think there's many things happening in the years, not in five years, maybe in 20/30 years but this industry is big, this industry is endless.

Yeah, you are going to think I'm mad here, but I can see in 5/6/7 years' time that those that want to do it, they can have a chip inserted underneath the skin. That chip will be able to recognise total energy expenditure. It will recognise heart rate, it will recognise deficiencies of vitamins and minerals. Then the chip will be connected to an app on your phone that then detects okay, you know, James has fallen a little bit low on iron. So we're now going to recommend that he has an iron-based meal, but the app will be connected to your oven and your fridge or whatever.

**Mohamed:** That's crazy how this industry may change, you know, especially now when you were talking, it came to my mind this artificial intelligence. Now, the AI industry can do everything for you. You can just sit there and watch; how capable is that? Me as a nutritionist, I will use the AI and I will give it two or three main pieces of information and it does the whole meal plan, the whole programme for the athletes. So yeah, man, it's crazy how the technology is improving. The technology is big, will be a big part in our industry which is sports nutrition. I believe it's getting there and it will be booming in the future and we never know how it will end.

**You said that you've got your console, your PlayStation, you read books, you read journals. Have you read a book recently that stands out that either influenced your practice or just one that you really enjoyed?**

**Mohamed:** Okay, if we speak about the nutrition industry, I haven't read any books recently; I mostly read online. But for books that will stand out, I believe there are two books that I love most. One is called *Atomic Habits* by James Clear. There is another one called *Deep Work*, by Cal Newport. Yeah, I love that book. So these are the last two books that I read. But the book that has really influenced me big time is called *The Laws of Human Nature* by Robert Greene. I love his books. Robert Greene books are amazing. I have all his series; it changes the way you think and changes the way you behave. They change the way you look at the world and look at people.

**You strike me as a man who is energetic, you're front facing, you're in sixth gear all the time, which is great because it's attractive and it's engaging. What do you do that keeps you like this every single day? What are your key principles?**

**Mohamed:** That's a good question. See, all of us are humans and I believe sometimes we feel down, sometimes we feel we are not energised, and that's fine. I don't believe I need something to motivate me. No, I need to build discipline. So that's why I love the book *Atomic Habits*; it's taught me how to build a habit from zero, from atomic habits, very small until it becomes one of the main things you do every day as a discipline.

So I believe I build a discipline that keeps me going as much as possible. When I wake up in the morning, I wake up, first thing I do, I just open my eyes, wash my face, hit the gym, I go to the gym directly. I train hard. I come back, take my post-workout meal, I come to my office, and I start to check what I have today. I have couple of hours that I study. I read for a couple of hours. By the way something I didn't mention is I have an online academy; it is called Arab Academy for Sports Nutrition. It's the only academy that speaks Arabic. I started it one year ago and it has around 13,000 students from all over the Arab countries. I do courses; they're like three to five-hour courses about sports nutrition and different sports. So I work on this academy; every month I have a new course or workshop online. So I work on that; I check out my clients. From there, I just start the day at that time, and then have a break. What do I have to do in the break, I do something entertainment, PlayStation, I just play, I just enjoy my time. I have to give myself a break. Then I'll go to the family. I'll come back again. I keep working. So I don't push myself all the time so I don't get bored and I don't feel frustrated. No, I have to give myself breaks. So I believe when I go to do my workout in the morning, I feel really energised; the day I don't do that, man, I don't feel as much as when I work out.

If I have any time left, I do my social media posts. That's it, that's how I structure my day. I don't have something that I do as a job. Everything is online. Unless I have to travel with my athletes, I do everything online. So the office that you see now, it's my home which most of the time I'm in. I just go sleep and come back. So yeah, that's in general how it goes.

**So in your experience what makes a successful nutritionist?**

**Mohamed:** Success in my opinion is not just being good at what you do as work or as a job. But success comes in many different ways. It's really important to be successful. You be good at what you do. You have to know what you're doing based on what. So you have this critical thinking, you'll be analytical about the things you're doing but at the same time, you have to be influential. I always say that you have to be influential to be successful. If you're not influential, you will not reach there. You have to understand how to speak, work on the body language, how to get there, network with people, get to know more people; the more people you know, especially people in your industry that will lift you up, the more you have the opportunity to succeed. Don't just stay like as an individual. We are creatures that have been created to be in groups. So the more you'll be with people that are in your industry, people who can help you think, can push you, the more they will give their time. So get there, build your network, build your character, work on the way you speak, the way you present yourself, the way you look also is important to me.

So try to be smart about how to get involved in each group that you believe will help, will lift you up. Also work or think out of the box. Don't just sit and believe nutrition is just what you read. How can I get there? Where are my opportunities?

Is it just in Bahrain now? Why shouldn't I think about Saudi, Dubai? How did this guy get successful? Look at them. Why does this guy have many athletes? What makes him outstanding? Study people. I believe that if we study people, and we study humans, we will get there as well. Because I always hear that from people; they say if you want to succeed, you have to fail. No, I don't have to fail. I have learned from the people who failed already. So they'll give me a shortcut anyway. But we'll have to wait until I fail on something. Let me study people, how they succeed, what failure they had, so I can go over it. So I believe it's really important for us to build ourselves and learn from others and get involved in groups that will help our network and our influence. I've never met anyone in our industry, to be honest, that worked so hard, and pushed themselves to the absolute limit and kept going and didn't succeed. It just can't be. Consistency is key.

So get there, work on yourself. Develop yourself. The most important asset that you have is your mind; work on it. Believe in yourself, keep learning. I always say be sceptical but open-minded. Whatever information you hear, listen to it; you may learn something. Sometimes I see these guys who are posting on social media they are so keen on evidence-based knowledge and I believe that it's okay, I'm a person that believes in evidence-based science. But when someone like let's say a bodybuilder speaks and says something, they may say he is just a bodybuilder not a scientist, but hey no! Listen, maybe you will get at least two or three words that make sense, and you gain knowledge you didn't know. So always listen. Whoever will come to me tells me, hey, you don't know if I will teach you something. No problem. Tell me. Let me listen to you. Why not? I may learn something new. So yeah, I believe we have to work on ourselves. We have to listen more. We have to work in our network and I believe if we keep at it and we are consistent with it, we will be successful.

## JAMES'S THOUGHTS

A standout moment in the interview with Mohamed is when he talks about social media being the power. If you are reading this book, it is because you saw it on Amazon organically, or it is probably because you saw me speak about it, advertise it or promote it on social media!

Social media is the biggest worldwide advertisement vehicle. And it is free! If you have your own business and are not using social media that well, then you need to start to!

I like how Mohamed talks about luck being opportunity when it meets preparation. I have personally experienced this many times.

Move faster... this is a great section of the interview and Mohamed has nailed it. How many of us wish we had started volunteering younger, posted more a few years ago, generated more experience with private clients many moons ago.

There is an old saying, the best time to plant an oak tree is 500 years ago, the next best is now. Linked to this, Mohamed finishes with success being linked to consistency and habits; work on yourself and keep developing yourself.

## CONCLUSION:
## *HOW TO STAND OUT FROM THE CROWD*

In book 1, I ended with the importance of understanding the trust equation. I won't go over that again now, but this still stands true for me every day.

Since book 1, I have been fortunate enough to mentor over 30 different practitioners from all over the world (America to Australia to Romania to Saudi Arabia). I say fortunate because I genuinely learn from and come away from each of my calls so motivated and passionate for the industry of sport nutrition. Whether it's the intricacies of trying to deliver nutrition on zero budget, or the fine line of a world champion boxer making the weight safely, the excitement between both these calls is the same!

These calls also remind me of how many different situations practitioners of all levels experience every day and the importance of me remaining well read in several different areas so I can assist (where possible) during these discussions. I'm not an expert and I am still learning every day, but it does keep pushing me to stay inquisitive with the whole of sport science and not just nutrition for rugby, football or boxing!

Having spent hundreds of hours doing mentee calls and hosting global conferences and performance nutrition community webinars, there are some key themes, traits and behaviours that I see from practitioners which seem to allow them to develop, progress and grow quicker than others.

## 1. DON'T BE AFRAID TO ASK
If asked in the right way, no question is a stupid question. Those who have an inquisitive mindset and want to know the "why" tend to be the ones who will continue to learn and progress.

## 2. IF YOU DON'T ASK YOU DON'T GET
There will be many people and businesses right underneath your nose who will be able to assist with your nutritional strategy; you just don't know they are there! Secondly, if you don't ask them to help then they don't know you want help. A case study example from me is our coffee supplier at Bristol Bears – Clifton Coffee. Since building a strong friendship between the club and the owner, they have provided us with about £10,000 RRP of coffee machines for free. All we do is buy the coffee beans from them. They were over the moon they could help us out.

## 3. YOU HAVE CLIENTS RIGHT IN FRONT OF YOU
If you haven't heard of Alex Hormozi and you are trying to run your own business, then get to know him quickly. Alex talks about how many clients are in your phone book; you have just forgotten about them. He calls it a scraping technique. Essentially, think about your inner circle of friends, family and phone contacts. How many of them know you have a business which offers a service, can help them achieve their goals, get them healthier? If they don't know about it, then you are not advertising well enough. Your first step is offering all of your family, friends and phone book your services before doing cold outreach. You will likely uncover a handful of clients straight away.

## 4. LEARN HOW TO BUILD RELATIONSHIPS WITH PEOPLE YOU HAVE NEVER MET!
As the late Dale Carnegie once said: "Remember that a person's name is to that person, the sweetest and most important sound in any language."

We have all been there; you have just met someone. You then see them again a few moments later but can't remember their name! Over recent years (and reminded by Dr David Dunne recently) I try to make a conscious effort to note down people's names. I don't have a great memory in the first place and so doing this simple task can help me a lot. It also means a lot to those you work with and especially in applied practice. For example, instead of keep saying "Chef" when you need something, say "Gareth"! It builds that relationship a lot quicker and easier.

Also, whether you are being parachuted into a boxing camp for the final two weeks of a massive fight or have started a new position at an organisation, your ability to build relationships with your team is going to be instrumental in your success in that camp or organisation.

**5. ENJOY THE PROCESS OF NETWORKING**
Networking is the process of making connections and building relationships.

Think about it, making connections. Life is all about making connections and the more connections you have the easier your career will be. The more people you can phone to ask for a favour, call in the car to reflect on your day and speak with to ask advice!

Building relationships: as humans we are social animals, we enjoy spending time with other humans and enjoy having social circles around us. Your career and your life are no different; building better relationships with the people you work with will ultimately make your job easier!

**6. SELF-DEVELOPMENT AND CONTINUAL DEVELOPMENT ARE CRUCIAL TO GETTING AHEAD OF YOUR PEERS**
Yes yes, well done, you have gone to university and obtained a degree. This does not automatically result in a career in sport. You must continually develop and push yourself to get better each week and each month. There is still so much I don't know about nutrition and sport science, but with an inquisitive mindset I am always looking to listen to the next podcast, read the recent review article or speak to others who are far more knowledgeable than me!

**7. TAKE ADVANTAGE OF TECHNOLOGY**
We are in the information age! The Information Age is the idea that access to and the control of information is the defining characteristic of this

current era in human civilisation. The Information Age – also called the Computer Age, the Digital Age and the New Media Age – is coupled tightly with the advent of personal computers.

If you don't take advantage of technology, computers, and artificial intelligence, you are going to get left behind!

**8. GAIN EXPERIENCE**
There are so many different opportunities. It annoys me when I hear people say they struggle to gain experience. There are so many opportunities to develop this experience in sport whether that be in the amateur, semi-professional or professional level. When was the last time you spoke to the owner of your local amateur boxing club, local Sunday league football team or local cross fit gym? These are brilliant places to start your journey of gaining experience and building relationships.

**9. I LOVE SEEING PRACTITIONERS TAKING INITIATIVE AND CRACKING ON**
This is a key trait difference I see between fast developers and slow developing practitioners. Having a level of initiative, "the ability to assess and initiate things independently", goes a long way in both business and sport. Are you someone that can think on your own feet or do you always need to have your hand held?

**10. TIME MANAGEMENT**
This is the most common theme that pops up in the weekly reflections from The Performance Nutrition Network. I often get asked, how do you manage to fit in Bristol Bears, boxers, high net worth individuals, writing a book, podcasts, running your own business, dog walks, gym, family time, relaxing time, corporate clients etc.

The honest answer, I haven't cracked it fully. There are times when the spinning of plates becomes too much, and I have to sacrifice one aspect to be able to do the other. But I'm getting better at time management every month. The idea of time blocking has helped a lot recently. Time blocking is a time management method that requires you to divide your day into blocks of time. Each block is dedicated to accomplishing a specific task or group of tasks, and only those specific tasks.

# FIND OUT MORE ABOUT THE PERFORMANCE NUTRITION NETWORK

To access the community, scan this QR code:

I specifically designed this community for practitioners who are keen to advance their careers. Our network thrives on a symbiotic relationship where mentorship is central – offering invaluable resources, insights and one-on-one guidance from seasoned professionals in the field of performance nutrition. Whether you're looking to refine your coaching techniques, delve deeper into scientific research, or understand the nuances of athlete engagement, our collective expertise is here to assist you in reaching your professional aspirations.

I believe that mentorship is not a one-way street but a collaborative effort that benefits all. As members, you will not only receive guidance but are also encouraged to share your own experiences, challenges and successes. This creates a cycle of continuous learning and improvement for everyone involved. Your active participation enriches the community, turning it into a dynamic and invaluable hub for career development in the realm of performance nutrition.

We are pleased to offer a dedicated space for you to learn, develop and thrive with other performance nutritionists.

*Our mission is to be the world's number 1 performance nutrition community, and we are committed to hosting a space where our actions align with our vision and purpose.*

Working with a big team of nutritionists would make growing your own personal business a lot easier.

Assurance, time-saving templates, educating athletes with confidence and progressing as a practitioner are all factors which are taken care of in the community.

Whether it's understanding how to negotiate a pay rise, how to put together an education curriculum, working with chefs, travel nutrition overseas or injury nutrition templates, the community has you covered. I have either shared my own content or other members have shared theirs.

In recent months we have had members apply to leading nutrition roles in sport and be successful, land applied PhD roles in elite level sport, and increase their monthly earnings by systemising their businesses, to name just a few.

I look forward to seeing you in the community soon.
James

# MENTORSHIP MOMENTS COURSE

To access the course, scan the below QR code:

Embark on a transformative mentorship journey with my premier course tailored for emerging nutrition coaches. Gleaned from a decade of experience in the performance nutrition industry, this course presents unmatched insights, including my work with elite rugby and football players, the establishment of supplement protocols for international football teams and guidance to championship-winning boxers.

Through exclusive video tutorials, you will delve into the intricate details of the profession, from effective networking to developing a distinctive vision.

As you grow and thrive, inspire those around you. By mastering the nuances of performance nutrition, become the role model whom budding nutritionists aspire to emulate.

Don't just move, soar. With the mentorship and tools at your disposal, fast-track your journey to the top echelons of the nutrition coaching world.

An outline of the modules included in the course is below:

**Module 1: Building Your Foundation (7 Lessons)**
Empower through clear vision, set actionable goals, meet athletes at their knowledge level, embrace reading & research, and understand that mere degrees don't suffice; self-reflection is key.

**Module 2: Expanding Your Expertise (6 Lessons)**
Attend essential conferences, meet players at their level, offer athlete reassurance, foster healthy food relationships, prioritise evidence-informed practice, and harness AI technology.

**Module 3: Career Development Strategies (6 Lessons)**
Seek guidance, foster strong relationships, master networking, leverage insights from experienced peers, understand the trust equation, and champion clear, abundant communication.

**Module 4: Establishing Your Reputation (5 Lessons)**
Boost reputation via social media; weigh Instagram vs. Twitter; create a personal website; strategic planning is vital; identify and promote your unique selling point.

**Module 5: Securing Opportunities (7 Lessons)**
Navigate job applications; be wary of Dunning-Kruger effect; remember all beginnings; learn from real-life job acquisition in sports; recognise nutritionist job scope; prioritise SENR registration and its specialist groups.

**Bonus Lessons!**

As I navigate the world of performance nutrition I will add key updated training videos to the course. These will be based on my own career progression but also key themes which crop up from within The Performance Nutrition Network. This means you get access to new videos each month!

# RECOMMENDED RESOURCES

Listed in order of mention

## BOOKS

*Who Not How: The Formula to Achieve Bigger Goals Through Accelerating Teamwork*, Dan Sullivan with Dr Benjamin Hardy

*The Infinite Game: How Great Businesses Achieve Long-lasting Success*, Simon Sinek

*Leaders Eat Last: Why Some Teams Pull Together and Others Don't*, Simon Sinek

*Zero to One: Notes on Start Ups, or How to Build the Future*, Peter Thiel with Blake Masters

*Peak: The New Science of Athletic Performance*, Dr Marc Bubbs

*Coaching for Performance: The Principles and Practice of Coaching and Leadership*, Sir John Whitmore

*Nudge: Improving Decisions about Health, Wealth and Happiness*, Richard Thaler and Cass R. Thunstein

*Range: How Generalists Triumph in a Specialized World*, David Epstein

*Will It Make The Boat Go Faster? Olympic-winning Strategies for Everyday Success*, Ben Hunt-Davis and Harriet Beveridge

*Being Mortal: Illness, Medicine and What Matters in the End*, Atul Gawande

*Madam Secretary*, Madeleine Albright

*Atomic Habits: An Easy & Proven Way to Build Good Habits & Break Bad Ones*, James Clear

*Deep Work: Rules for Focused Success in a Distracted World*, Cal Newport

*Kellie*, Kellie Harrington with Roddy Doyle

*Out Of Thin Air: Running Wisdom and Magic from Above the Clouds in Ethiopia*, Michael Crawley

*The Score Takes Care of Itself: My Philosophy of Leadership*, Bill Walsh, Steve Jamison and Craig Walsh

*Exercised: The Science of Physical Activity, Rest and Health*, Daniel Lieberman

*Burn: The Misunderstood Science of Metabolism*, Herman Pontzer

*Lessons in Chemistry*, Bonnie Garmus

*The Four Agreements: A Practical Guide to Personal Freedom*, Don Miguel Ruiz

*The Laws of Human Nature*, Robert Greene

## OTHER RESOURCES

The High-Performance podcast (Susie Ma)

The Ben Ryan podcast (Ben Ryan)

*The Last Dance* (Netflix documentary)

Leave Your Mark podcast (Scott Livingston)

The Eisenhower Matrix (created by President Dwight Eisenhower)

TickTick (todo list, checklist and task manager app)

Blinkist (book summarising app/subscription)

# ABOUT THE AUTHOR

We learnt about James's background in book 1. From his many months travelling, to his studies in Liverpool for his PhD and elements of his applied work.

Since book 1, James has continued his work in professional sport and with elite athletes from mainly football, rugby, boxing and combat sport and currently works as the lead nutritionist with Bristol Bears Rugby.

Over recent years, notably he was part of the Red Roses Women's Rugby team for 18 months and in that time, they won back-to-back Six Nations Championships. Regarding boxing, he has been part of Chris Billam-Smith's rise to winning the recent World Championship belt and also completed successful camps with Chris Eubank Jr, Harlem Eubank and rising star Adam Azim.

With a view to keep getting better, James has invested in his own mentor and business coach in Dan Lawrence and has joined him in business with Perform 365, a globally recognised performance support service for high net worth individuals and CEOs across the world.

Finally, James has successfully launched The Performance Nutrition Network, a fast-growing community of nutrition practitioners across the globe.

www.ingramcontent.com/pod-product-compliance
Lightning Source LLC
Chambersburg PA
CBHW051541020426

42333CB00016B/2037